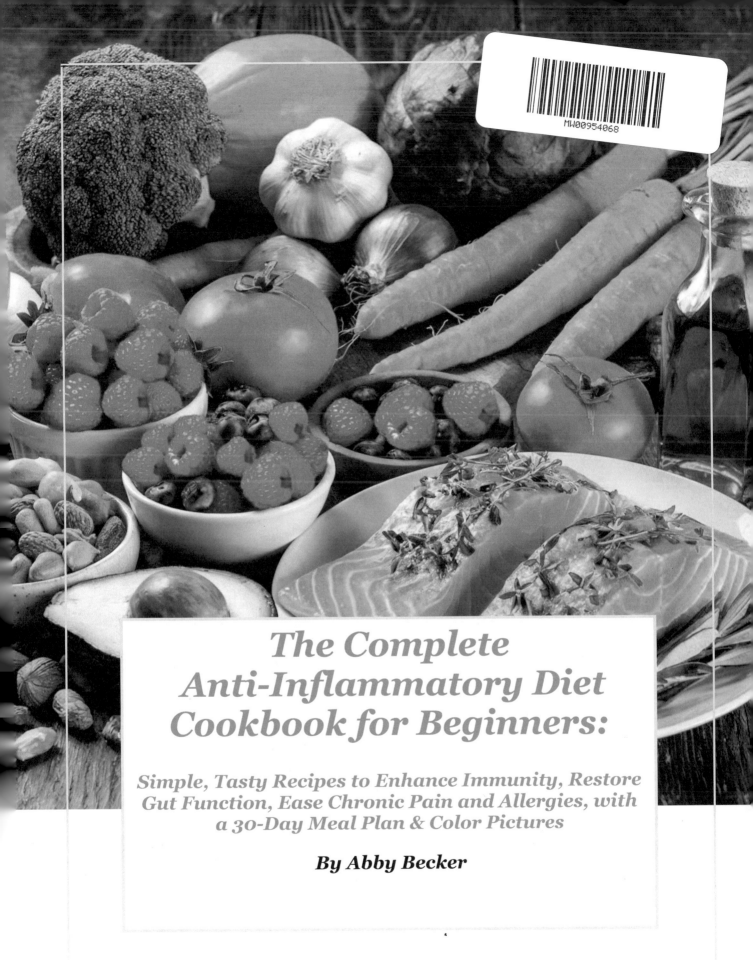

The Complete Anti-Inflammatory Diet Cookbook for Beginners:

Simple, Tasty Recipes to Enhance Immunity, Restore Gut Function, Ease Chronic Pain and Allergies, with a 30-Day Meal Plan & Color Pictures

By Abby Becker

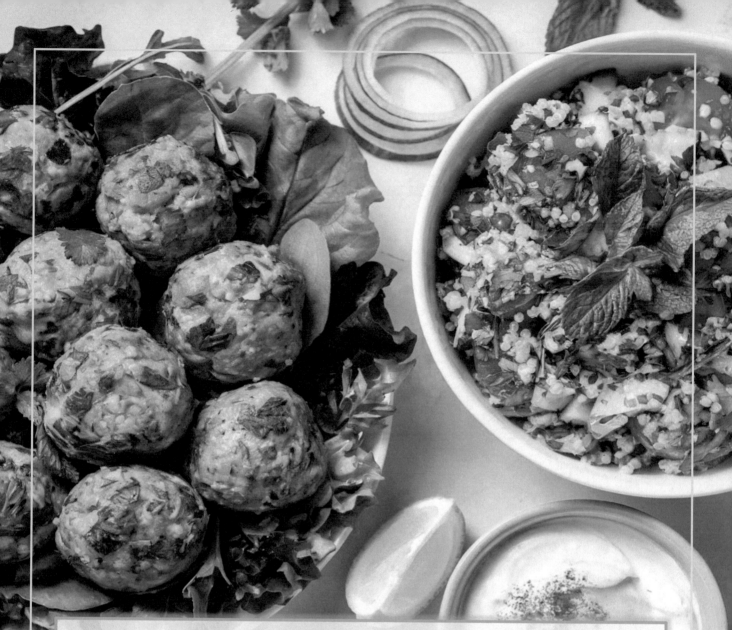

Friendly Disclaimer

Dear Reader, We're delighted you've chosen this cookbook. It's filled with recipes we believe you'll enjoy. Just a friendly reminder—while we've made every effort to offer you excellent tips and recipes to help reduce inflammation and improve your overall health, this book is not a substitute for professional medical advice. It's important to consult with your healthcare provider about your diet, especially if you have specific health concerns. Our recipes are crafted to inspire you and bring joy to your culinary adventures while supporting your journey to better health.

Please remember that the path to improving health and managing inflammation is unique for everyone. What works for one person may not work for another. Therefore, treat this book as a guide and a companion on your journey, always listening to your body and the advice of your healthcare team. Let's embark on this flavorful adventure towards well-being together!

Abby Becker

Table of Contents

Welcome, Dear Reader!

If you're holding this book, you've already taken the first step toward improving your health. Congratulations on making this important decision! I am confident that together, we can walk this path step by step—from understanding the basics of an anti-inflammatory diet to confidently applying it in your life, enhancing your well-being, boosting your energy levels, and feeling a renewed sense of vitality.

My name is Abby Becker, and I am a practicing dietitian-nutritionist. My main goal is to help people maintain their health and prevent serious illnesses through dietary changes and the adoption of restorative diets.

This topic became deeply personal to me when my mother was diagnosed with type 2 diabetes at the age of 55, and later, my son was diagnosed with type 1 diabetes. These events prompted me to explore deeply the subject of nutrition and its impact on health.

Numerous medical and scientific studies show that one of the causes of diabetes, as well as many other serious diseases, is chronic hidden inflammation in the body. In this book, I aim to provide information that will help you neutralize this process and even reverse it through a balanced anti-inflammatory diet.

I understand that changing dietary habits and a lifestyle that has been developed over years, or even generations, is not easy. But having walked this path—which, in the end, is not as daunting as it seems at first—you will feel rejuvenated, brimming with strength and energy, and grateful to yourself for having made this choice. Every positive change in your routine and diet is an investment in your healthy future. Take a step, and the path will appear!

So, let's set off on this journey!

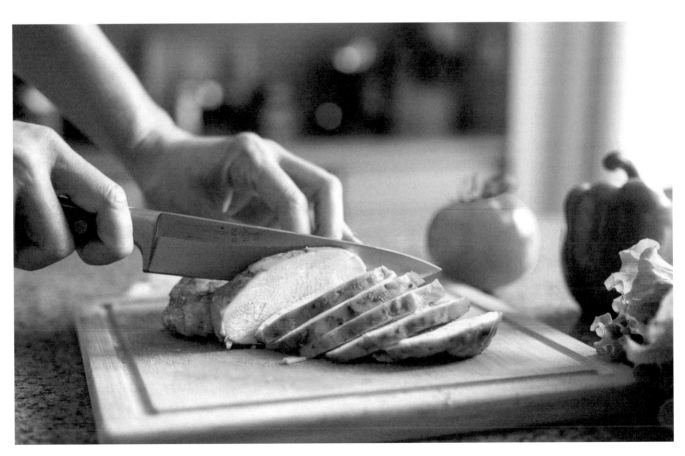

The Anti-Inflammatory Diet: History, Key Concepts, and Principles

The concept of the anti-inflammatory diet has garnered significant attention in recent decades, as scientists and medical professionals have increasingly explored the link between chronic inflammation and the development of serious diseases. While the idea that diet affects health has been known for thousands of years (as seen in traditional medical practices like Ayurveda and Chinese medicine), modern science has substantially refined and expanded this understanding.

In the mid-20th century, there was a surge in research focused on the causes of chronic diseases such as cardiovascular disease, diabetes, and cancer. Researchers began to observe that inflammation frequently accompanies these conditions, even if it does not present overtly.

During the 1970s and 1980s, scientists made significant breakthroughs in understanding how the immune system functions and how inflammation is related to its response to various stimuli. This led to the realization that chronic inflammation can arise not only from infections but also from various factors such as stress, poor diet, and environmental pollution.

By the 1990s, research began to highlight that certain foods could either exacerbate or alleviate inflammation. These studies examined the impact of saturated fats, trans fats, sugar, and processed foods on the body. Concurrently, scientists started investigating the benefits of omega-3 fatty acids, antioxidants, and other nutrients that may help reduce inflammation levels.

By the early 2000s, the anti-inflammatory diet started to gain popularity among doctors, dietitians, and the general public. It has been the subject of numerous books and articles. Today, the anti-inflammatory diet is considered one of the key tools for maintaining health, preventing chronic, age-related diseases, and slowing premature aging. It is based on foods rich in healthy fats, antioxidants, and fiber, which help reduce inflammation levels in the body and support overall well-being.

Let's delve deeper into the key aspects.

What is Inflammation?

Inflammation is the body's natural protective response to injury or infection. It plays a crucial role in helping our body fight off harmful microorganisms and repair damaged tissues. The primary goal of inflammation is to restore homeostasis, or balance, within the body. Therefore, inflammation itself is not always harmful; its impact depends on the type and duration of the inflammation.

Acute Inflammation is the body's initial, short-term response to injury or infection, usually lasting from a few hours to a few days. The main signs of acute inflammation include redness, heat, swelling, pain, and sometimes loss of function in the affected area. These symptoms are related to increased blood flow and the migration of immune cells to the site of injury to combat the threat.

Stages of Acute Inflammation:

1. Initiation:
When tissues are damaged, inflammatory mediators such as histamines, prostaglandins, and cytokines are released. These substances increase blood flow to the affected area, causing redness and heat in the region.

2. Recruitment:

Leukocytes (white blood cells), including neutrophils and macrophages, are recruited to the site of injury or infection. These cells actively destroy pathogens and clear away debris from damaged tissues.

3. Resolution:

Once the threat has been neutralized, anti-inflammatory mechanisms are activated to halt the inflammatory process. At this stage, tissue repair and healing begin.

Let's break this down with a simple example.

Imagine you accidentally cut your finger with a kitchen knife.

First, you feel pain and notice your finger starting to turn red and swell. This immediate response is the initiation stage, where your body sends 'alarm signals' in the form of inflammatory mediators, which increase blood flow to the site of the injury. Your finger might feel a bit warm to the touch—another sign that blood is actively rushing to the wound to help immune cells reach the area as quickly as possible.

Next, leukocytes—tiny "soldiers"—come into action, destroying any bacteria that might have entered the wound and clearing away damaged cells. Your finger might swell a bit because the immune cells are actively fighting off potential infection.

Finally, once the danger has passed, the inflammation begins to subside. Your finger stops hurting and swelling, and the skin starts to heal. This healing process is the "resolution" stage, where the body begins to return to its normal state.

However, if acute inflammation does not eliminate the threat, or if the body is continually exposed to harmful factors, inflammation can become chronic.

Chronic Inflammation

Chronic inflammation is a hidden threat that can go unnoticed for years, causing no apparent symptoms. However, it gradually takes a destructive toll on the body.

Characteristics of Chronic Inflammation:

- **Continuous Tissue Damage:** Prolonged inflammation leads to continuous destruction of cells and tissues, which can eventually cause severe organ damage.

- **Fibrosis and Scarring:** Chronic inflammation promotes the formation of scar tissue and fibrosis, reducing the functionality of affected organs.

- **Altered Immune Response:** Ongoing inflammation can disrupt the normal functioning of the immune system, triggering the development of autoimmune diseases and diminishing the body's ability to fight infections.

Impact of Chronic Inflammation on Health

While acute inflammation is the body's natural protective response, chronic inflammation becomes a destructive process that undermines health.

Low-grade, chronic inflammation is one of the primary causes of many serious diseases:

- **Cardiovascular diseases** (Atherosclerosis, Ischemic heart disease, Heart failure, Hypertension)

- **Neurodegenerative diseases** (such as Alzheimer's disease, Parkinson's disease, and Multiple sclerosis)

- **Autoimmune disorders** (Rheumatoid arthritis, Systemic lupus erythematosus, Scleroderma, Autoimmune thyroiditis, Type 1 diabetes)

- **Various cancers** (Liver cancer, Stomach cancer, Colorectal cancer, Pancreatic cancer, Lung cancer, Bladder cancer, Cervical cancer)

Overall, about 60-70% of all deaths worldwide are associated with diseases caused by chronic inflammation.

Chronic inflammation can go unnoticed for a long time, as it does not cause the vivid symptoms that acute inflammation does. However, certain signs may indicate its presence in the body and should prompt concern:

1. **Chronic Fatigue:** A constant feeling of tiredness, even after adequate rest.

2. **Muscle and Joint Pain:** Experiencing pain in muscles or joints without a clear reason may be related to inflammation.

3. **Digestive Issues:** Inflammation can manifest through symptoms like bloating, discomfort, or irritable bowel syndrome.

4. **Frequent Colds and Infections:** A weakened immune system caused by chronic inflammation can lead to frequent infections.

5. **Skin Changes:** Acne, rashes, redness, or other skin eruptions can be signs of inflammatory processes in the body.

6. **Weight Gain:** Gaining excess weight, especially in the abdominal area, can also be linked to chronic inflammation.

7. **Mood Issues:** Depression, anxiety, and other mood changes may result from inflammatory processes.

8. **Brain Fog:** Difficulty concentrating, memory problems, or feeling "foggy-headed" may also be associated with hidden inflammation.

If you notice any of the symptoms listed above, it is a good idea to consult a doctor for a thorough examination. To detect hidden inflammatory processes, several tests are frequently utilized, including:

1. **C-Reactive Protein (CRP):** This is one of the most common markers of inflammation. The CRP level in the blood increases during inflammation, including chronic inflammation. A high-sensitivity CRP test (hs-CRP) can detect even low levels of inflammation, making it useful for assessing the risk of cardiovascular diseases.

2. **Erythrocyte Sedimentation Rate (ESR):** This is a classic and widely available test that also helps detect inflammation. Although it is less specific than CRP, ESR remains a useful indicator of the overall inflammatory state in the body.

3. **Fibrinogen:** This protein is involved in blood clotting and can increase during inflammation. Elevated fibrinogen levels are associated with an increased risk of cardiovascular diseases and may indicate chronic inflammation.

4. **Interleukin-6 (IL-6):** This cytokine plays a key role in regulating inflammatory processes. Elevated IL-6 levels may indicate the presence of inflammation.

5. **Homocysteine Levels:** High levels of this substance in the blood can be associated with inflammation and an increased risk of cardiovascular diseases.

6. **Cytokine Levels and Other Inflammatory Markers:** In more specific cases, doctors may order tests for various cytokines and other markers, such as tumor necrosis factor-alpha (TNF-α).

These tests help doctors assess the presence and level of hidden chronic inflammation, which is important for determining the next steps in treatment and disease prevention.

Factors That Cause Hidden Chronic Inflammation in the Body

Years of medical research have shown that certain factors can disrupt the body's homeostasis and contribute to the development of inflammation:

1. **Unhealthy Diet.**

A diet high in processed foods, sugar, trans fats, and fatty meats is one of the primary contributors to hidden inflammation. These foods can trigger an inflammatory response, disrupting the delicate balance between pro-inflammatory and anti-inflammatory molecules in the body. Additionally, a lack of antioxidants, omega-3 fatty acids, and fiber in the diet exacerbates inflammation, as these substances play a key role in suppressing it. In the following sections, we will explore in detail which foods to include in your diet and which to avoid to reduce inflammation. After all, the main theme of our book is precisely how to maintain health and manage inflammation through proper nutrition.

2. **Obesity.**

Excess weight, particularly when it involves the accumulation of fat around internal organs (visceral fat), poses a serious health risk because it is closely linked to chronic inflammation. Visceral fat tissue in the abdominal area not only stores fat but also actively releases substances such as cytokines and other pro-inflammatory molecules, which trigger inflammatory processes throughout the body. When visceral fat becomes excessive, it turns into a constant source of inflammation. This chronic inflammation slows down metabolism, reduces insulin sensitivity, and can contribute to the development of various diseases, such as type 2 diabetes and cardiovascular diseases. This creates a vicious cycle: inflammation promotes weight gain, and excess weight, in turn, sustains and amplifies inflammatory processes, further deteriorating health.

3. **Chronic Stress.**

Stress is not only a psychological burden but also a powerful trigger of inflammation. Constant emotional or physical tension stimulates the production of stress hormones, such as cortisol. Initially, cortisol helps regulate the inflammatory response, but prolonged stress keeps cortisol levels elevated for extended periods. Over time, this can lead to a state of cortisol resistance, akin to insulin resistance.

When cells lose sensitivity to cortisol, despite its high levels, they do not receive the signals needed to suppress inflammatory processes. This leads to a state where inflammation in the body increases, despite the presence of cortisol. Such resistance can be a cause of chronic inflammation.

4. Toxic Exposure.

Our environment is filled with potential sources of toxins that can cause inflammation, and modern lifestyles only exacerbate their impact on our bodies. Polluted air containing fine particles of harmful substances (soot, metals, organic chemicals, pollen), tobacco smoke, alcohol, industrial chemicals, and pesticides all affect body cells, causing damage and activating inflammatory responses. And the list doesn't end there. One of the key sources of toxins in our lives is plastic. Everyday items, ranging from food packaging to cosmetics, often contain chemicals such as bisphenol A (BPA) and phthalates, which can leach into our bodies. These substances disrupt the endocrine system and can lead to inflammatory processes, affecting various organs and systems. In the long term, constant exposure to toxins can weaken the immune system, making the body more vulnerable to infections and inflammatory diseases. Avoiding all these factors completely is impossible, but steps can be taken to minimize them, such as reducing plastic use, quitting smoking, limiting alcohol consumption, and choosing environmentally friendly products. Taking care of your environment is an important step toward reducing inflammation in the body and maintaining overall health.

5. Lack of Physical Activity.

A sedentary lifestyle is associated with elevated levels of inflammatory markers, such as C-reactive protein (CRP) and interleukin-6 (IL-6), which contribute to chronic inflammation. In contrast, physical activity helps regulate inflammation and reduces the risk of developing chronic diseases. Regular exercise decreases inflammatory markers and improves insulin sensitivity. It also boosts the body's antioxidant systems and reduces fat tissue, a source of pro-inflammatory cytokines.

6. Infections and Chronic Conditions.

Certain infections and chronic conditions can maintain low levels of inflammation in the body. For example, diseases such as chronic viral infections or periodontitis (gum inflammation) can contribute to the persistence of the inflammatory process.

7. Chronic Sleep Deprivation.

Lack of sleep or poor sleep quality significantly impacts inflammatory processes in the body. During sleep, the body recovers and regulates many physiological functions, including the immune response. Chronic sleep deprivation results in elevated levels of inflammatory markers, including C-reactive protein (CRP) and interleukin-6 (IL-6), which can provoke and sustain inflammatory processes. Lack of sleep can also disrupt circadian rhythms, further contributing to immune system regulation imbalances. Sleep deficiency and poor sleep quality can impair the body's resistance to stress, increasing the production of cortisol and other stress hormones, which in turn amplifies inflammation. This creates a vicious cycle where lack of sleep leads to increased inflammation, and inflammation worsens sleep quality. Additionally, studies show that chronic sleep deprivation may be associated with increased sympathetic nervous system activity and decreased parasympathetic nervous system activity, leading to elevated blood pressure and inflammatory responses. Thus, sufficient and high-quality sleep is critically important for maintaining healthy levels of inflammatory markers and preventing chronic inflammation.

All these factors that cause hidden inflammation are closely interwoven and affect our bodies in a complex manner. Each factor contributes in its own way to sustaining the inflammatory process, and achieving health and well-being requires considering all of them. However, since this is, after all, a cookbook, let's focus on what we can change immediately—our diet.

"You are what you eat" — this quote perfectly captures the importance of nutrition in our lives. Nutrition is not just fuel for the body; it's a key factor that influences our health and even our genes. Scientific studies demonstrate that diet can influence gene expression, thereby affecting the risk of developing various diseases.

A well-balanced diet should supply all the essential nutrients, including vitamins, minerals, micronutrients, proteins, fats, carbohydrates, and fiber. Vitamins like C, D, and E, and minerals such as zinc and selenium, play crucial roles in supporting the immune system and combating oxidative stress. Omega-3 fatty acids are vital for cardiovascular health, while fiber promotes normal bowel function and prevents constipation.

An inadequate intake of these nutrients can lead to deficiencies, which, in turn, can cause various health problems. A lack of vitamins and minerals can weaken the immune system, increase the risk of chronic diseases, slow down metabolism, and even affect cognitive functions. Therefore, it is important to maintain a balanced and diverse diet to support health and well-being.

Secrets of Anti-Inflammatory Eating: What to Eat and How to Prepare for Optimal Health

Unlike certain dietary regimens, such as the keto diet, the DASH diet, or the carnivore diet, an anti-inflammatory diet is not about the strict exclusion of any food group. It is based on a balanced approach that includes all the main macronutrients—proteins, fats, and carbohydrates—in their most beneficial forms.

The main principle of an anti-inflammatory diet is to include foods that help reduce inflammation in the body and exclude those that can increase inflammation and worsen overall health.

The Dietary Inflammatory Index (DII) and the Dietary Inflammation Score (DIS) are valuable tools in this context. These indices are designed to assess how specific foods or an overall diet contribute to or reduce inflammatory processes in the body. Foods with negative values on these indices have anti-inflammatory properties, while foods with positive values may promote inflammation.

Below is a list of foods with negative DII and DIS values that possess strong anti-inflammatory properties. These ingredients should form the foundation of your daily diet to effectively soothe inflammation and strengthen your health.

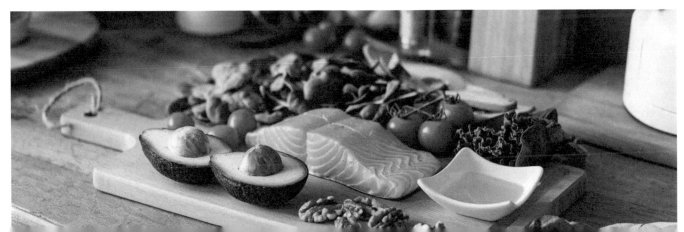

Anti-Inflammatory Foods (What to Include in Your Diet)

Food Group	Examples	Benefits
Leafy Greens and Cruciferous Vegetables	Various cruciferous vegetables (broccoli, Brussels sprouts, white cabbage, red cabbage, cauliflower), lettuce (iceberg, head, leaf), spinach, parsley, arugula, kohlrabi, watercress	Contain antioxidants and polyphenols that activate a specific protein called Nrf2. This protein helps protect cells from oxidative stress and inflammation, playing a key role in maintaining overall health.
Tomatoes	Tomatoes, tomato juice, tomato sauces and paste, salsa	These foods are classified into a separate group due to their high anti-inflammatory properties. They contain β-carotene, vitamin C, and lycopene, one of the most potent antioxidants.
Fruits and Berries	Fresh fruits (apples, pears, pineapples, kiwi, lemon, grapefruit, oranges, apricots, mango) and berries (strawberries, raspberries, blueberries, cherries, grapes, watermelon, melon), as well as natural juices made from them	Contain flavonoids that suppress the production of pro-inflammatory cytokines and are powerful antioxidants.
Vegetables and Fruits with Deep Yellow or Orange Color	Melon, peaches, apricots, carrots, dark yellow or orange squash, figs	Rich in provitamin A carotenoids, such as β-carotene and α-carotene, which are potent antioxidants.

Other Vegetables	Vegetables not listed above and root vegetables (e.g., okra, bell peppers, onions, zucchini, eggplants, asparagus, beets, radishes, turnips, sweet potatoes), mushrooms	These vegetables are rich in antioxidants, polyphenols, vitamins C and E, and beta-carotene, which help neutralize free radicals and reduce inflammation in the body.
Legumes	Green beans, peas, lima beans, lentils, and other legumes (excluding soy)	High in folate, iron, and isoflavones, and possess significant antioxidant activity; also rich in fiber, which supports beneficial changes in the gut microbiota.
Fish	Tuna, salmon, other light and dark meat fish, breaded fish cakes or fish sticks	Contain omega-3 fatty acids that suppress pro-inflammatory processes in the body.
Lean Poultry	Chicken, turkey, quail	Contain low levels of saturated fats and L-arginine, which improves endothelial function and reduces inflammatory processes.
Pungent Vegetables	Garlic, onions, green onions, leeks, ginger	These vegetables not only add rich flavor to dishes but also actively protect the body against chronic inflammation due to their high content of antioxidants, phytonutrients, and sulfur compounds.

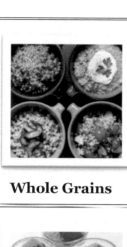 **Whole Grains**	Oats, buckwheat, wild rice, barley, quinoa, pearl barley, millet	An excellent source of fiber, B vitamins, minerals (such as magnesium, iron, and zinc), and antioxidants. They help regulate blood sugar levels, support healthy digestion, and contribute to reducing inflammation.
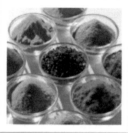 **Herbs and Spices**	Turmeric, cinnamon, black pepper, red pepper, cloves, rosemary, cilantro, dill, saffron, tarragon, thyme	Help reduce inflammation in the body due to their antioxidant and antibacterial properties, support improved metabolism, and maintain immune system function.
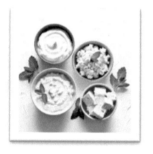 **Low-Fat Dairy Products**	Milk, yogurt, probiotic-fermented cheese, cottage cheese, ricotta	Contains calcium, which reduces oxidative damage in the intestines; dairy fat contains fatty acids with potential anti-inflammatory properties. Probiotics support the balance of gut microbiota, which helps reduce the production of pro-inflammatory cytokines and improve gut barrier function, reducing systemic inflammation.
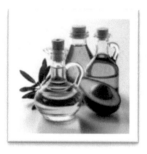 **Healthy Oils**	Olive oil (extra virgin), avocado oil, flaxseed oil, walnut oil, coconut oil (in moderation)	These oils are rich in healthy fats, such as monounsaturated and polyunsaturated fatty acids, as well as omega-3s and antioxidants, which help reduce inflammation in the body.
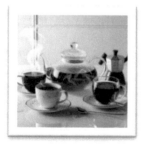 **Coffee and Tea**	Coffee, herbal tea, black tea, green tea	Tea contains flavonoids and antioxidants (such as epicatechin and quercetin); coffee contains phytochemicals and antioxidants. Herbal teas contain natural antioxidants and phytochemicals.

Foods that Promote Inflammation (What to Avoid)

Food Group	Examples	Effects
 Refined Sugar and High-Glycemic Index Foods	Refined sugar, sugary drinks, sweet snacks, confectionery, candies	Causes sharp fluctuations in blood glucose levels, which can lead to inflammation. Disrupts metabolism, contributing to fat accumulation and obesity. Leads to insulin resistance and type 2 diabetes. Promotes calcium excretion from the body, weakening bones and leading to osteoporosis. Participates in the glycation process, which damages collagen fibers, making them stiff and less elastic, accelerating skin aging and worsening joint conditions.
 Fatty and Processed Meats	Fatty meats (beef, lamb, pork), lard, sausages, bacon, hot dogs, steaks	Contain saturated fats and compounds like nitrites and nitrates that can increase inflammation. Additionally, high-temperature cooking methods (frying, grilling) lead to the formation of advanced glycation end products (AGEs), which also promote inflammation.
 Trans Fats and Hydrogenated Oils, and Products Made with Them	Margarine, donuts, cookies, waffles, pastries, muffins, candies, crackers, chips, microwave popcorn, frozen pizza, processed snacks, fried fast foods	Raise "bad" cholesterol (LDL) levels and lower "good" cholesterol (HDL) levels, disrupting lipid balance in the body, increasing the risk of cardiovascular diseases, and triggering inflammatory reactions. Additionally, such foods can contribute to obesity and insulin resistance, further intensifying inflammatory processes in the body.
 Processed and Refined Foods, Fast Food	White bread, white rice, pasta, sugary cereals, confectionery, chips, fast food, soft drinks, sweet sauces, packaged juices, canned soups	Low in fiber, which disrupts normal bowel function and can lead to chronic inflammation in the gastrointestinal tract. They are quickly digested, causing sharp spikes in blood sugar levels, which may stimulate the production of inflammatory molecules and enhance inflammatory processes. Contain artificial colors, flavor enhancers, preservatives, and other chemical additives that can trigger inflammatory reactions in the body.

Food Group	Examples	Effects

Certain Types of Vegetable Oils | Soybean oil, corn oil, sunflower oil, safflower oil, canola oil | These oils are high in omega-6 fatty acids, which can disrupt the balance between omega-3 and omega-6 fatty acids in the body. When consumed in excess relative to omega-3s, omega-6 fatty acids can promote the formation of pro-inflammatory molecules, such as prostaglandins and leukotrienes, leading to increased inflammation in the body. |
|

Alcohol | Strong and low-alcohol drinks (wine, cognac, whiskey, rum, beer) in excessive amounts | Increases levels of inflammatory markers in the blood and causes oxidative stress, leading to cell damage. Disrupts the gut barrier function, increasing its permeability and allowing toxic substances to enter the bloodstream. Imbalances gut microbiota, promoting inflammation. Weakens the immune system, making it harder to combat inflammation. |

When discussing an anti-inflammatory diet, it is essential to emphasize the importance of adequate intake of plain water. Water is the foundation of life, supporting the normal functioning of all bodily systems, including the immune system. A lack of water can disrupt metabolism and increase the concentration of toxins, which in turn can exacerbate inflammatory processes.

Moreover, water helps flush out harmful substances and excess sodium, both of which can contribute to inflammation. Maintaining optimal hydration levels can improve blood circulation, reduce swelling, and support joint health. Therefore, regular water consumption should be an integral part of an anti-inflammatory diet and a healthy lifestyle, promoting your overall health and well-being.

These are the basic principles of an anti-inflammatory diet, which can significantly improve your health. However, it's important to remember that each body is unique, and individual needs can vary. For example, many people today have intolerances to dairy products or gluten and are susceptible to various allergic reactions to different foods.

Gluten is a protein found in wheat, rye, barley, and all derivatives of these grains (bulgur, couscous, pearl barley, barley groats, semolina, pasta). For people with increased sensitivity to gluten—which currently includes about 30% to 50% of the population—these foods trigger an inflammatory response in the gut, which can lead to intestinal lining damage, impaired nutrient absorption, and increased inflammation throughout the body. I am not referring to celiac disease, which affects about 1% of the global population, but rather to various manifestations of intolerance, which can appear as bloating, fatigue, headaches, and skin rashes. Therefore, if you notice that certain gluten-containing foods cause discomfort, you should consider eliminating them from your diet and consulting a specialist. Replacing wheat, rye, and barley with gluten-free alternatives can help reduce inflammation levels and improve overall well-being.

A similar situation exists with dairy products. The term "lactose intolerance" is widely known, and various issues with lactose digestion are observed in 50-75% of the world's population. Entire shelves in stores are dedicated to lactose-free dairy products. However, not everyone knows that many people suffer from intolerance not to lactose (milk sugar), but to one of the milk proteins, particularly casein. Lactose-free alternatives will not help them. Clinical signs of this condition can include skin manifestations (itchy rash, eczema, dermatitis), gastrointestinal symptoms (abdominal pain, vomiting, diarrhea, bloating, and constipation), and sometimes respiratory symptoms (cough, choking attacks, rhinitis). If you suspect a milk protein intolerance, it may be necessary to temporarily eliminate animal-derived dairy products and replace them with plant-based alternatives, such as almond, coconut, or oat milk.

The problem is further complicated by the fact that with chronic intestinal inflammation, complex proteins like casein and gluten (which have a glue-like consistency) are highly likely to eventually become non-digestible and act like toxins, triggering a new cycle of inflammation.

Foods such as eggs, seafood, and soy are excellent sources of high-quality protein and essential vitamins and minerals that support overall health. They are not on the restricted list. However, it's important to note that these foods can cause allergic reactions in a significant number of people. Therefore, their consumption requires caution, especially for those prone to allergies.

It is important to be attentive to your body and monitor which foods cause negative symptoms so you can eliminate them promptly and prevent harmful processes in the body.

Vitamins: Allies in the Fight Against Inflammation

This chapter would be incomplete without discussing the essential vitamins needed to maintain health and combat inflammation. The key vitamins include A, C, D, E, and the B group.

Vitamin A
Sources: Carrots, sweet potatoes, pumpkin, spinach, eggs.
Vitamin A can be obtained from animal sources (liver, fish oil, eggs), while its precursor, beta-carotene, comes from plant sources (carrots, apricots, sweet potatoes, pumpkin, spinach). Vitamin A helps maintain the integrity of mucous membranes and skin, which is crucial for protecting the body from pathogens. It also plays a key role in regulating the immune system. A deficiency in vitamin A can lead to reduced immunity, vision problems, and slowed tissue regeneration.
Recommended dosage: Adults are advised to consume around 700-900 mcg of vitamin A per day. This vitamin is usually obtained in sufficient amounts from food, but supplements may be needed in cases of deficiency. Dosage should be determined by a healthcare professional, as overdose can be toxic.

Vitamin C
Sources: Citrus fruits, kiwi, strawberries, cherries, sea buckthorn, black currants, broccoli, cabbage, red bell pepper.
Vitamin C is a powerful antioxidant that neutralizes free radicals and reduces inflammation in the body. It also plays a role in collagen synthesis, which is important for joint and skin health. A deficiency in vitamin C can weaken the immune system, increase susceptibility to infections, and slow wound healing.
Recommended dosage: Adults are recommended to consume 100 mg of vitamin C per day, but in cases of active inflammation or stressful situations, the requirement may increase. For anti-inflammatory effects, a daily intake of 500-1000 mg of vitamin C is recommended.

Vitamin D

Sources: Fatty fish (salmon, sardines), egg yolks, mushrooms, leafy greens, cheese.

Vitamin D regulates immune responses and has strong anti-inflammatory effects. It also plays a crucial role in maintaining bone health. A deficiency in vitamin D can lead to chronic inflammation, weakened bones and muscles, and an increased risk of autoimmune diseases.

Recommended dosage: For most people, a daily intake of 600-800 IU (International Units) of vitamin D is recommended, but those with a deficiency, especially in northern latitudes, may require additional supplementation, with dosage determined individually based on blood tests.

Vitamin K2

Sources: K2 is found in animal products like meat, eggs, cheese, butter, and some fermented foods.

Vitamin K2 plays an important role in the absorption of vitamin D and its effectiveness in the body. Vitamin D aids in calcium absorption, while vitamin K2 helps direct this calcium to the bones and teeth, preventing its accumulation in the arteries and soft tissues, which can lead to calcification and an increased risk of cardiovascular diseases. The combined action of vitamins D and K2 ensures proper calcium distribution, strengthens bone tissue, and supports cardiovascular health. A deficiency in vitamin K can disrupt this process, reducing the effectiveness of vitamin D and increasing the risk of diseases related to calcium imbalance.

Recommended dosage: The exact dosage of vitamin K2 is not yet established, but generally, 90-120 mcg per day is recommended. In cases of K2 deficiency, supplementation may be required, especially in the presence of chronic inflammation.

Vitamin E

Sources: Nuts, seeds, avocados, and vegetable oils (especially olive oil).

Vitamin E protects cells from oxidative stress and has anti-inflammatory effects. A deficiency in vitamin E can lead to cell membrane damage and increased inflammation.

Recommended dosage: The daily requirement for vitamin E is about 15 mg. If there is a deficiency, it is recommended to include foods rich in this vitamin in the diet or take supplements.

Omega-3 Fatty Acids

Although not vitamins, omega-3 fatty acids deserve special mention for their strong anti-inflammatory properties. They are found in fatty fish (salmon, sardines), flaxseeds, and walnuts. A lack of omega-3s in the diet can lead to increased inflammation and worsening overall health.

Recommended dosage: The daily requirement for omega-3 fatty acids is approximately 250-500 mg, but in cases of chronic inflammation, a higher dosage may be required, usually achieved through supplementation.

Looking at the impressive list of foods with anti-inflammatory properties that form the basis of our diet, you can see that it can be diverse and delicious. It's not about restrictions. All restrictions and beliefs are in our minds. We may think that life won't be enjoyable without a favorite treat, but it's just a matter of habit and awareness. A dietary habit can be formed in 14 days. If you go without sweets for two weeks, you may find you don't crave them anymore. As someone with issues digesting gluten and dairy, I can tell you that living without these products is easy! Much easier than living with headaches, constant fatigue, and facial breakouts. Easier, healthier, more energetic, and just as tasty!

I hope I haven't tired you too much with the theoretical part. I want you to not just blindly follow some rules, but to do so consciously and with an understanding of the processes happening in your body, fully aware of the consequences of your dietary changes.

Now, let's put on our aprons and good moods and embark on our healthy and delicious journey!

US to Metric and UK Cooking Measurement Conversions

US Measurement	Metric Equivalent
1 teaspoon (tsp)	5 ml
1 tablespoon (tbsp)	15 ml
1 cup	240 ml
1 pint	473 ml
1 quart	946 ml
1 ounce (oz)	28 g
1 pound (lb)	454 g
1 pound (lb)	454 g
1 gallon	3.785 liters
1 fluid ounce (fl oz)	30 ml

Oven Temperatures

Temperature (°F)	Temperature (°C)
250°F	120°C
275°F	135°C
300°F	150°C
325°F	160°C
350°F	175°C
375°F	190°C
400°F	200°C
425°F	220°C
450°F	230°C

Kitchen Conversion Chart

Cups	Oz	G	Tbsp	Tsp	Ml
1/16	1/2	15	1	3	15
1/8	1	50	2	6	50
1/4	2	60	4	12	60
1/3	3	70	5	16	70
1/2	4	115	8	24	125
2/3	5	140	11	32	150
3/4	6	170	12	36	175
1	8	225	16	48	250

BREAKFASTS: A DELICIOUS START TO THE DAY

Veggie-Stuffed Omelet
A light and nutritious breakfast featuring eggs, packed with high-quality protein, and seasonal vegetables

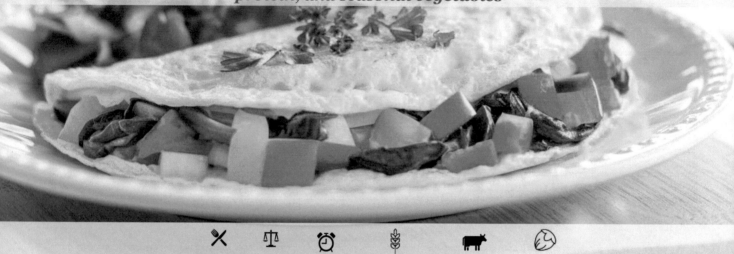

✕	⚖	⏰	🌾	🐄	🌍
2 svgs.	10 min.	10 min.	Gluten-Free	Dairy-Free	Nut-Free

Ingredients:
- 4 large eggs
- 1/4 cup chopped bell peppers (red and yellow)
- 1/4 cup diced onions
- 1/4 cup chopped spinach
- 1/4 cup chopped tomatoes
- 2 tablespoons chopped fresh herbs (such as parsley or chives)
- Salt and pepper to taste
- 1 tablespoon olive oil

Instructions:
1. Prepare the Egg Mixture: In a bowl, whisk the eggs with a pinch of salt and pepper until smooth. Divide the mixture into two equal portions.
2. Sauté the Vegetables: Heat 1/2 tablespoon of olive oil in a non-stick skillet over medium heat. Add the bell peppers and onions, and sauté until softened, about 3 minutes. Add the spinach and tomatoes, cooking just until the spinach wilts. Remove the vegetables from the skillet and set aside.
3. Cook the First Omelet: Add a small amount of the remaining olive oil to the skillet. Pour in one portion of the whisked eggs, tilting the pan to ensure an even layer. Cook without stirring until the eggs are mostly set but still slightly runny on top, about 3-4 minutes.
4. Add Vegetables and Fold: Evenly distribute half of the sautéed vegetables over one half of the omelet. Fold the other half of the omelet over the vegetables and cook for another minute to fully set the eggs. Slide the omelet onto a plate.
5. Repeat for the Second Omelet: Repeat steps 3 and 4 with the second portion of the egg mixture and the remaining vegetables.
6. Garnish and Serve: Garnish each omelet with fresh herbs and serve immediately.

Nutritional Information: *250 calories, 14g protein, 8g carbohydrates, 18g fats, 2g fiber, 370mg cholesterol, 220mg sodium, 300mg potassium.*

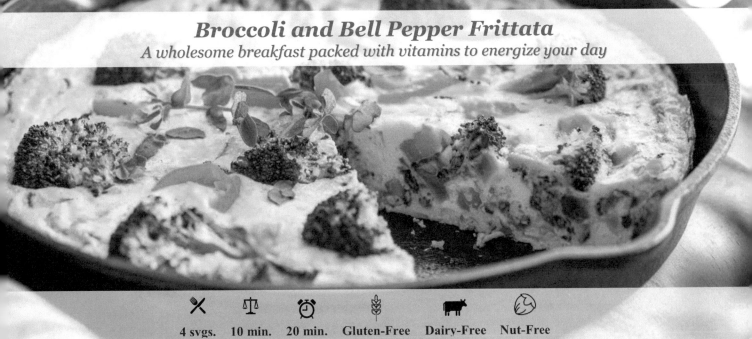

Broccoli and Bell Pepper Frittata
A wholesome breakfast packed with vitamins to energize your day

4 svgs.   10 min.   20 min.   **Gluten-Free**   **Dairy-Free**   **Nut-Free**

Ingredients:
- 6 large eggs
- 1/2 cup unsweetened almond milk (or any other non-dairy milk)
- 1 cup broccoli florets, chopped
- 1 red bell pepper, diced
- 1/2 cup onion, finely chopped
- 1/4 cup dairy-free cheese (optional)
- 1 tablespoon olive oil
- Salt and pepper to taste
- Fresh herbs for garnish (such as parsley or chives)

Instructions:
1. Preheat Oven: Preheat your oven to 350°F (175°C).
2. Sauté Vegetables: In a large, oven-safe skillet, heat the olive oil over medium heat. Add the chopped onion, bell pepper, and broccoli. Sauté for about 5-7 minutes, until the vegetables are softened.
3. Prepare the Egg Mixture: In a large bowl, whisk together the eggs, almond milk, salt, and pepper until well combined. Stir in the dairy-free cheese if using.
4. Combine and Cook: Pour the egg mixture over the sautéed vegetables in the skillet. Let it cook on the stovetop for 2-3 minutes until the edges start to set.
5. Bake: Transfer the skillet to the preheated oven and bake for 10-12 minutes, or until the frittata is fully set and slightly golden on top.
6. Serve: Garnish with fresh herbs and serve warm. Slice into wedges and enjoy a healthy, protein-packed meal.

Nutritional Information: *220 calories, 14g protein, 8g carbohydrates, 15g fats, 3g fiber, 370mg cholesterol, 200mg sodium, 350mg potassium.*

Acai Smoothie Bowl

An energizing and nutritious breakfast, rich in protein and fiber.

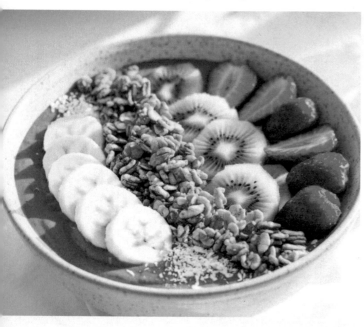

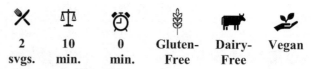

🍴	⚖️	⏰	🌾	🐄	🌱
2 svgs.	**10 min.**	**0 min.**	**Gluten-Free**	**Dairy-Free**	**Vegan**

Ingredients:

- 1 packet (about 100g) frozen acai puree
- 1 ripe banana, sliced
- 1/2 cup frozen mixed berries (blueberries, strawberries, raspberries)
- 1/2 cup unsweetened almond milk (or any other plant-based milk)
- 1 tablespoon chia seeds (optional, for added fiber)
- 1/2 cup granola (gluten-free or nut-free, if needed)
- Fresh fruit slices (such as banana, kiwi, or strawberries) for topping
- 1 tablespoon shredded coconut (optional)
- Honey or maple syrup for drizzling (optional)

Instructions:

1. Blend the Smoothie Base: In a high-speed blender, combine the frozen acai puree, half of the banana, frozen mixed berries, almond milk, and chia seeds (if using). Blend until smooth and thick, scraping down the sides as needed.
2. Assemble the Smoothie Bowl: Divide the smoothie mixture between two bowls. It should be thick enough to hold toppings without sinking.
3. Add Toppings: Arrange the remaining banana slices, granola, fresh fruit slices, and shredded coconut on top of each smoothie bowl. Drizzle with honey or maple syrup if desired.
4. Serve: Enjoy immediately, savoring the vibrant flavors and crunchy texture of this anti-inflammatory breakfast or snack.

Nutritional Information: *300 calories, 5g protein, 50g carbohydrates, 10g fats, 9g fiber, 0mg cholesterol, 60mg sodium, 350mg potassium.*

Notes:

Acai *berries are packed with antioxidants and have been shown to reduce oxidative stress and inflammation. Combined with fiber-rich bananas and crunchy granola, this smoothie bowl is not only delicious but also a great way to start your day with anti-inflammatory benefits.*

Tip:

In the Snacks section, you'll find a recipe for wholesome homemade granola, allowing you to control every ingredient for the perfect, healthy mix tailored to your taste.

Green Smoothie with Spinach, Avocado, and Kiwi

A nourishing smoothie that promotes hydration and boosts immunity.

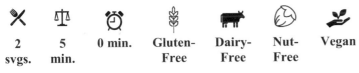

X	⚖	⏰	🌾	🐄	🌰	🌱
2 svgs.	5 min.	0 min.	Gluten-Free	Dairy-Free	Nut-Free	Vegan

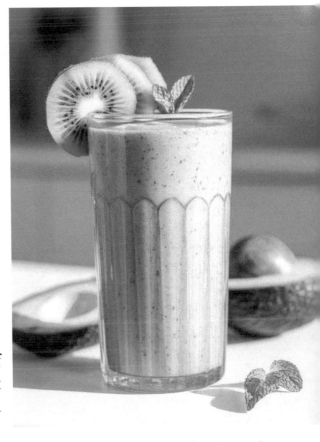

Ingredients:

- 1 ripe avocado, peeled and pitted
- 2 ripe kiwis, peeled and sliced
- 2 cups fresh spinach leaves
- 1 banana (optional, for added sweetness)
- 1/2 cup coconut water or plain water
- Juice of 1/2 lime
- A few ice cubes (optional, for a chilled smoothie)

Instructions:

1. Combine all ingredients in a blender.
2. Blend on high speed until smooth and creamy. If the smoothie is too thick, add a bit more coconut water or plain water to reach the desired consistency.
3. Taste and adjust the sweetness by adding a little more banana or a splash of maple syrup if desired.
4. Serve immediately, garnished with a slice of kiwi or a sprinkle of chia seeds if you like.

Nutritional Information: *240 calories, 3g protein, 35g carbohydrates, 12g fats, 9g fiber, 0mg cholesterol, 20mg sodium, 800mg potassium.*

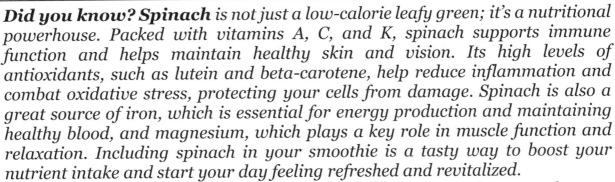

__Did you know? Spinach__ is not just a low-calorie leafy green; it's a nutritional powerhouse. Packed with vitamins A, C, and K, spinach supports immune function and helps maintain healthy skin and vision. Its high levels of antioxidants, such as lutein and beta-carotene, help reduce inflammation and combat oxidative stress, protecting your cells from damage. Spinach is also a great source of iron, which is essential for energy production and maintaining healthy blood, and magnesium, which plays a key role in muscle function and relaxation. Including spinach in your smoothie is a tasty way to boost your nutrient intake and start your day feeling refreshed and revitalized.

__Tip:__ Feel free to experiment by adding cucumber, parsley, lettuce, celery, or apple to this green smoothie for extra freshness and nutrition. Smoothies like this are an excellent way to increase your vegetable and fiber intake, making it easy to incorporate more greens into your diet. Don't hesitate to get creative with your favorite veggies!

Berry Chia Oatmeal with Old-Fashioned Oats

A fiber-rich breakfast boosted with antioxidants from fresh berries and omega-3 fatty acids.

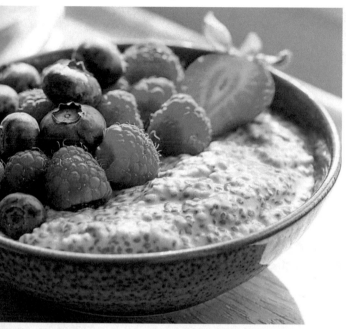

✗	⚖	⏱	🌾	🐄	🌍	🌱
2 svgs.	5 min.	10 min.	Gluten-Free	Dairy-Free	Nut-Free	Vegan

Ingredients:

- 1 cup old-fashioned oats
- 2 cups water or unsweetened almond milk
- 1/2 cup fresh mixed berries (blueberries, raspberries, strawberries)
- 1/4 cup chia seeds
- 1 tablespoon maple syrup (optional)
- 1/2 teaspoon vanilla extract
- Pinch of salt

Instructions:

1. In a medium saucepan, bring water or almond milk to a boil. Add the old-fashioned oats and a pinch of salt, then reduce the heat to a low simmer.

2. Cook the oats, stirring occasionally, for about 10-15 minutes until they are tender and have absorbed most of the liquid.

3. Stir in chia seeds and vanilla extract, and continue to cook for another 2-3 minutes to allow the chia seeds to swell and the mixture to thicken.

4. Remove from heat. If a sweeter taste is desired, stir in the maple syrup.

5. Serve the oatmeal in bowls, topped with fresh berries.

Nutritional Information: *315 calories, 11g protein, 48g carbohydrates, 11g fats, 16g fiber, 0mg cholesterol, 30mg sodium, 210mg potassium.*

Notes:

Old-fashioned *oats, or rolled oats, are less processed than quick oats, retaining a heartier texture, richer flavor, and a lower glycemic index, which helps manage blood sugar levels and reduce inflammation. They're rich in soluble fiber, particularly beta-glucan, which lowers cholesterol and supports heart health. Oats also provide essential vitamins and minerals, such as manganese, magnesium, phosphorus, B vitamins, and iron, promoting energy, digestion, and overall well-being. Adding oats to your diet offers sustained energy and numerous health benefits.*

Tip:

This recipe is easily adaptable to any seasonal berries or fruits. You can also top it with nuts for added crunch, as long as there are no allergies.

Buckwheat Pancakes with Apple Sauce

A gluten-free twist on traditional pancakes served with a fragrant homemade apple sauce.

✕	⚖	⏰	🌾	🐄	🌍
4 svgs.	**10 min.**	**20 min.**	**Gluten-Free**	**Dairy-Free**	**Nut-Free**

Ingredients:

For the buckwheat pancakes:
- 1 cup buckwheat flour
- 1 tablespoon ground flaxseed (optional, for extra fiber)
- 1 tablespoon baking powder
- 1/4 teaspoon salt
- 1 tablespoon maple syrup or honey
- 1 1/4 cups almond milk or other plant-based milk
- 1 teaspoon vanilla extract
- 1 tablespoon coconut oil, melted (plus extra for cooking)
- 2 large eggs

For the apple sauce:
- 3 medium apples, peeled, cored, and chopped
- 1/4 cup water
- 1 tablespoon maple syrup or honey
- 1/2 teaspoon ground cinnamon
- 1/4 teaspoon ground ginger (optional)
- 1/2 teaspoon lemon juice

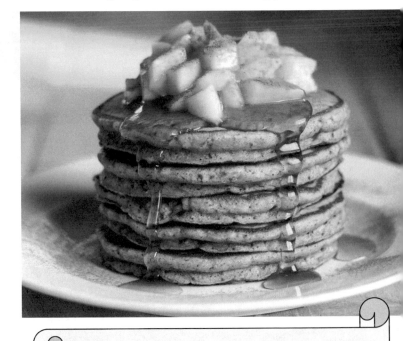

Buckwheat is naturally gluten-free and rich in antioxidants like rutin, which helps reduce inflammation and improve blood circulation. It is also a great source of high-quality protein, containing all essential amino acids, making it a fantastic option for muscle health and overall body repair.

Instructions:

1. **Prepare the Apple Sauce:** In a medium saucepan, combine the chopped apples, water, maple syrup, cinnamon, and ginger. Bring to a simmer over medium heat and cook for about 10-15 minutes, stirring occasionally, until the apples are soft. Remove from heat, stir in lemon juice, and mash the apples to your desired consistency. Set aside.

2. **Prepare the Buckwheat Pancakes:** In a large bowl, whisk together the buckwheat flour, ground flaxseed, baking powder, and salt. In a separate bowl, whisk the eggs, almond milk, maple syrup, vanilla extract, and melted coconut oil until well combined. Pour the wet ingredients into the dry ingredients and gently stir until just combined. Be careful not to overmix, as this can make the pancakes tough.

3. **Cook the Pancakes:** Heat a non-stick skillet or griddle over medium heat and lightly grease with coconut oil. Pour about 1/4 cup of the batter for each pancake onto the skillet. Gently spread the batter into a circular shape if needed to form a pancake.

4. Cook until bubbles form on the surface and the edges look set, about 2-3 minutes. Flip and cook for another 2-3 minutes until golden brown and cooked through. Repeat with the remaining batter.

5. **Serve:** Stack the buckwheat pancakes on plates and generously spoon the warm apple sauce over the top. Garnish with a sprinkle of cinnamon or a drizzle of maple syrup if desired.

Nutritional Information: *290 calories, 8g protein, 40g carbohydrates, 10g fats, 6g fiber, 110mg cholesterol, 150mg sodium, 250mg potassium.*

Avocado and Salmon Toast

A heart-healthy breakfast rich in healthy fats, combining creamy avocado with omega-3-rich salmon for a delicious and nutritious start to your day.

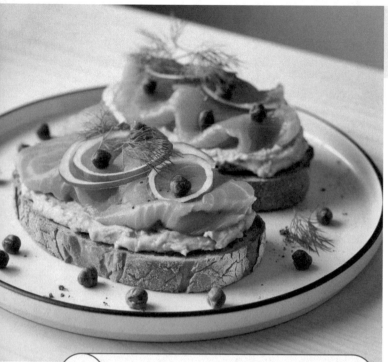

✗	⚖	⏰	🌾	🐄	🌰
2 svgs.	5 min.	2 min.	Gluten-	Dairy-Free	Nut-Free

Ingredients:

- 2 slices of gluten-free bread
- 1 ripe avocado, peeled and mashed
- 4 oz cured salmon
- 1 tablespoon lemon juice
- Salt and black pepper to taste
- 1/4 red onion, thinly sliced
- Fresh dill for garnish
- 1 tablespoon capers (optional)

Instructions:

1. Toast the slices of gluten-free bread until golden and crispy, either in a toaster or a dry frying pan.
2. In a small bowl, mix the mashed avocado with lemon juice, salt, and black pepper.
3. Spread the avocado mixture evenly on each slice of toasted bread.
4. Arrange the cured salmon slices over the avocado.
5. Top with sliced red onion, capers (if using), and a sprinkle of fresh dill.
6. Serve immediately, enjoying the creamy texture of the avocado with the fresh flavor of the salmon.

Nutritional Information: *310 calories, 18g protein, 20g carbohydrates, 20g fats, 7g fiber, 22mg cholesterol, 640mg sodium, 550mg potassium.*

***Salmon** is rich in omega-3 fatty acids, which help reduce inflammation and support heart health. It also provides high-quality protein and essential vitamins like D and B12, which strengthen the immune system and maintain healthy bones. Plus, it's a great source of selenium, an antioxidant that protects cells, and potassium, which helps regulate blood pressure. So, if you're still not a fan of salmon, it's time to make amends. Your body will thank you!*

***Avocado** is packed with heart-healthy monounsaturated fats that help lower bad cholesterol levels. It's also rich in fiber, which aids digestion, and contains vitamins C, E, K, and B-6, along with folate and potassium, which support overall health. This creamy fruit not only enhances the flavor of your toast but also boosts its nutritional value.*

Berry and Nut Yogurt Parfait with Honey

- *A delightful combination of creamy yogurt, fresh berries, crunchy nuts, and a drizzle of honey, creating a perfect balance of textures and flavors for a satisfying start to your day.*

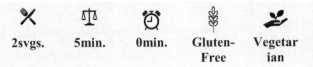

✗	⚖	⏰	🌾	🌿
2svgs.	5min.	0min.	Gluten-Free	Vegetarian

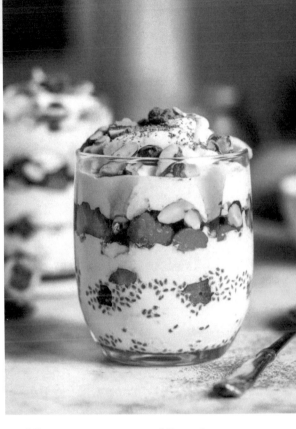

Ingredients:
- 1 cup Greek yogurt
- 1/4 cup mixed nuts (such as almonds, walnuts, and pecans), chopped
- 2 tablespoons honey (or maple syrup for a vegan option)
- 1/2 cup fresh berries (such as blueberries, strawberries, or raspberries)
- 1 tablespoon chia seeds (optional, for extra fiber and omega-3s)
- 1/2 teaspoon ground cinnamon

Instructions:
1. Layer the Parfait: In each serving glass, spoon a layer of Greek yogurt at the bottom.
2. Add Nuts and Berries: Sprinkle a layer of chopped nuts and fresh berries over the yogurt.
3. Repeat Layers: Add another layer of yogurt, followed by more nuts and berries.
4. Drizzle with Honey: Drizzle honey (or maple syrup) over the top of each parfait.
5. Garnish: Sprinkle with chia seeds and a pinch of cinnamon for extra flavor and nutrition.
6. Serve: Enjoy immediately, or refrigerate for a quick, nutritious snack later.

Nutritional Information: *280 calories, 12g protein, 28g carbohydrates, 14g fats, 5g fiber, 10mg cholesterol, 50mg sodium, 350mg potassium.*

Notes:

Greek yogurt is an excellent addition to an anti-inflammatory diet. It is rich in protein, which helps maintain muscle mass and supports overall health, and contains probiotics, beneficial bacteria that promote a healthy gut, reduce inflammation, and enhance immune function. Greek yogurt is also a great source of **calcium, magnesium, potassium, iodine, phosphorus, and zinc**, which are essential for bone health, metabolic processes, and reducing inflammation. Additionally, it provides vitamins **B2 (riboflavin)** and **B12**, which are important for energy metabolism and nervous system health, as well as vitamins **A** and **D**, which support immune function and help combat inflammation.

Quinoa Porridge with Almond Milk and Cinnamon
An energizing and nutritious breakfast, rich in protein and fiber.

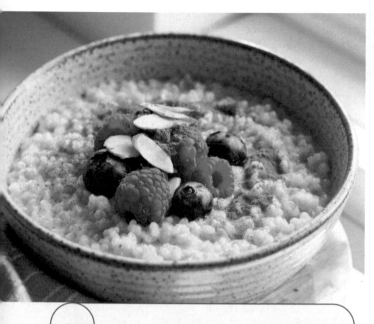

✕	⚖	⏰	🌾	🐄	🌍	🌱
2 svgs.	**5 min.**	**20 min.**	**Gluten-Free**	**Dairy-Free**	**Nut-Free**	**Vegan**

Ingredients:
- 1 cup quinoa, rinsed
- 2 cups unsweetened almond milk
- 1 tablespoon maple syrup or honey
- (optional)
- 1 teaspoon ground cinnamon
- 1/4 teaspoon vanilla extract
- Pinch of salt
- Optional toppings: fresh berries,
- sliced almonds, chia seeds, or additional cinnamon

Instructions:
1. **Cook the Quinoa:** In a medium saucepan, combine the rinsed quinoa and almond milk. Bring to a boil over medium heat, then reduce the heat to low, cover, and let it simmer for about 15 minutes, or until the quinoa is tender and has absorbed most of the liquid.
2. **Add Flavor:** Stir in the maple syrup or honey (if using), ground cinnamon, vanilla extract, and a pinch of salt. Continue to cook, stirring occasionally, for another 5 minutes until the porridge reaches your desired consistency.
3. **Serve:** Spoon the quinoa porridge into bowls and top with your favorite toppings, such as fresh berries, sliced almonds, chia seeds, or an extra sprinkle of cinnamon.
4. **Enjoy:** Serve warm and enjoy a comforting and nourishing breakfast.

Nutritional Information: *250 calories, 7g protein, 40g carbohydrates, 7g fats, 5g fiber, 0mg cholesterol, 150mg sodium, 450mg potassium.*

Notes:

Quinoa *is a true superfood due to its high content of folate, fiber, and plant-based protein. A cup of quinoa contains about 10–15 grams of protein, more than most grains, with a balance of essential amino acids comparable to milk proteins.*

It is also rich in minerals such as iron, calcium, zinc, phosphorus, potassium, magnesium, manganese, copper, and selenium. Quinoa is packed with vitamins, particularly B vitamins (such as B1, B2, B6, and folate), and also provides vitamin E, an antioxidant that helps protect cells from damage.

Quinoa is gluten-free, has a low glycemic index, and is easy to digest, making it suitable for people with diabetes or those looking to prevent it.

Additionally, quinoa contains both essential and non-essential amino acids, including lysine, which helps with calcium absorption and supports overall bone health.

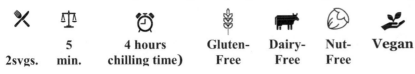

Chia Pudding with Mango and Coconut

This refreshing pudding is not only delicious but also packed with fiber, omega-3s, and vitamins, making it a perfect choice for a healthy breakfast or a light dessert.

✕ 2svgs.	⚖ 5 min.	⏰ 4 hours chilling time)	🌾 Gluten-Free	🐄 Dairy-Free	🌍 Nut-Free	🌱 Vegan

Ingredients:
- 1/4 cup chia seeds
- 1 cup unsweetened coconut milk
- 1 tablespoon maple syrup or honey (optional)
- 1/2 teaspoon vanilla extract
- 1 ripe mango, peeled and diced
- 1/4 cup shredded coconut (unsweetened)
- Fresh mint leaves for garnish (optional)

Instructions:

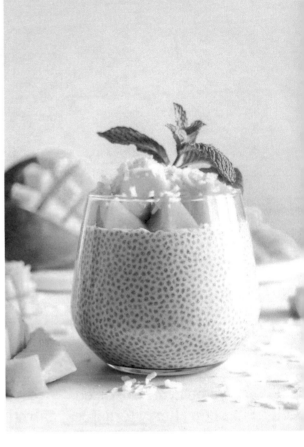

1. Prepare the Chia Pudding: In a medium bowl, whisk together the chia seeds, coconut milk, maple syrup (if using), and vanilla extract. Stir well to ensure the chia seeds are evenly distributed.
2. Chill: Cover the bowl and refrigerate for at least 4 hours, or overnight, until the chia seeds have absorbed the liquid and the mixture has thickened to a pudding-like consistency.
3. Assemble the Pudding: Once set, give the pudding a good stir and divide it evenly between two serving glasses or bowls. Top each serving with the diced mango and a sprinkle of shredded coconut.
4. Serve: Garnish with fresh mint leaves if desired, and enjoy this refreshing, anti-inflammatory treat.

Nutritional Information: *250 calories, 5g protein, 28g carbohydrates, 14g fats, 10g fiber, 0mg cholesterol, 30mg sodium, 380mg potassium.*

Notes:

Chia *seeds are tiny powerhouses of nutrition! They're loaded with essential minerals like iron, zinc, calcium, phosphorus, magnesium, and selenium—perfect for those looking to boost their nutrient intake, especially if you follow a vegetarian diet. Chia seeds are particularly rich in magnesium and calcium, which are key for bone health and muscle function.*

These little seeds are also packed with omega-3 fatty acids (ALA), known for their ability to help reduce inflammation and support heart health. Plus, chia seeds are full of antioxidants, like chlorogenic acid and caffeic acid, which help protect your body from oxidative stress.

And it doesn't stop there! Chia seeds contain vitamins such as B1 (thiamine), B3 (niacin), and E, as well as powerful phytonutrients like myricetin, quercetin, and kaempferol, all of which help keep your immune system in top shape.

Quinoa Salad with Avocado and Cherry Tomatoes
A nourishing salad is rich in protein and healthy fats.

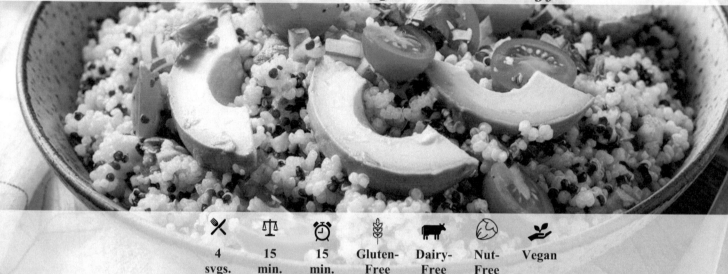

4 svgs.	15 min.	15 min.	Gluten-Free	Dairy-Free	Nut-Free	Vegan

Ingredients:
- 1 cup quinoa, rinsed
- 2 cups water
- 1 ripe avocado, diced
- 1 cup cherry tomatoes, halved
- 1/4 cup red onion, finely chopped
- 1/4 cup fresh cilantro or parsley, chopped
- 2 tablespoons extra virgin olive oil
- 1 tablespoon fresh lemon juice
- 1 tablespoon balsamic vinegar
- Salt and pepper to taste

Instructions:
1. Cook the Quinoa: In a medium saucepan, bring the water to a boil. Add the rinsed quinoa, reduce heat to low, cover, and simmer for about 15 minutes, or until the quinoa is tender and the water is absorbed. Fluff with a fork and let it cool.
2. Prepare the Salad: In a large mixing bowl, combine the cooked quinoa, diced avocado, halved cherry tomatoes, chopped red onion, and fresh cilantro or parsley.
3. Make the Dressing: In a small bowl, whisk together the olive oil, lemon juice, balsamic vinegar, salt, and pepper until well combined.
4. Assemble the Salad: Pour the dressing over the quinoa mixture and toss gently to combine. Taste and adjust seasoning as needed.
5. Serve: Serve immediately or refrigerate for a few hours to allow the flavors to meld. This salad can be enjoyed cold or at room temperature.

Nutritional Information: *320 calories, 7g protein, 28g carbohydrates, 22g fats, 6g fiber, 0mg cholesterol, 50mg sodium, 600mg potassium.*

Notes:

Quinoa *is not only a complete protein but also rich in magnesium and antioxidants, which help reduce inflammation. Avocado adds healthy monounsaturated fats, while cherry tomatoes provide vitamin C and lycopene, both of which have anti-inflammatory properties. This salad is a perfect, nutrient-dense choice for a light meal or side dish.*

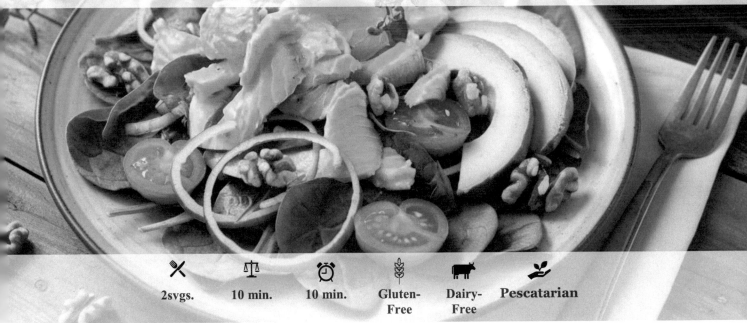

Salmon, Spinach, and Walnut Salad
A source of omega-3 fatty acids, vitamins, and minerals.

🍴	⚖️	⏰	🌾	🐄	🌱
2svgs.	10 min.	10 min.	Gluten-Free	Dairy-Free	Pescatarian

Ingredients:
- 4 oz cooked salmon fillet, flaked
- 4 cups fresh baby spinach leaves
- 1/4 cup walnuts, lightly toasted and chopped
- 1/2 avocado, sliced
- 1/4 red onion, thinly sliced
- 1/4 cup cherry tomatoes, halved
- 2 tablespoons extra virgin olive oil
- 1 tablespoon lemon juice
- 1 teaspoon Dijon mustard
- Salt and pepper to taste

Instructions:
1. Prepare the Salmon: If not already cooked, season the salmon fillet with salt and pepper, then pan-sear or bake at 350°F (175°C) for about 10 minutes, or until cooked through. Let it cool slightly, then flake the salmon into bite-sized pieces.
2. Assemble the Salad: In a large bowl, combine the fresh spinach leaves, flaked salmon, toasted walnuts, sliced avocado, red onion, and cherry tomatoes.
3. Make the Dressing: In a small bowl, whisk together the olive oil, lemon juice, Dijon mustard, salt, and pepper until emulsified.
4. Dress the Salad: Drizzle the dressing over the salad ingredients and toss gently to combine. Adjust seasoning to taste.
5. Serve: Serve immediately, enjoying the fresh flavors and crunchy textures of this nutritious, anti-inflammatory salad.

Nutritional Information: *350 calories, 20g protein, 12g carbohydrates, 27g fats, 6g fiber, 50mg cholesterol, 150mg sodium, 700mg potassium.*

Notes:

This salad combines the anti-inflammatory benefits of omega-3 rich salmon, vitamin-packed spinach, and antioxidant-laden walnuts. The healthy fats from the avocado and olive oil further support the body's ability to fight inflammation, making this salad a powerful ally in maintaining overall health.

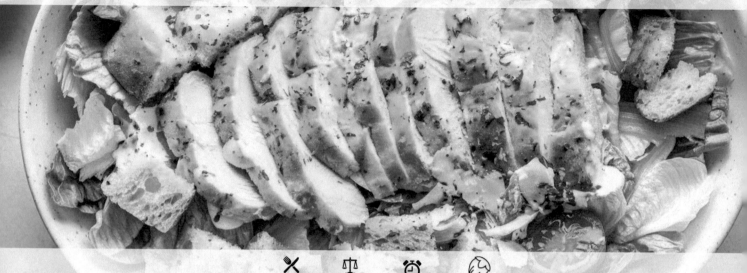

Chicken Caesar Salad with Homemade Croutons
A classic salad in a healthy version with a low-fat dressing.

4 svgs.   **15 min.**   **20 min.**   **Nut-Free**

Ingredients:
For the Salad:
- 2 cooked chicken breasts, sliced
- 6 cups romaine lettuce, chopped
- 1/4 cup grated Parmesan cheese (optional)
- 1/2 cup cherry tomatoes, halved (optional)
- 1/4 cup homemade croutons (see recipe below)

For the Croutons:
- 2 slices gluten-free bread, cut into cubes
- 2 tablespoons olive oil
- 1/2 teaspoon garlic powder
- 1/2 teaspoon dried oregano
- Salt and pepper to taste

For the Dressing:
- 1/4 cup plain Greek yogurt
- 1/4 cup mayonnaise (or more Greek yogurt for a lighter option)
- 2 tablespoons freshly squeezed lemon juice
- 1 teaspoon Dijon mustard
- 1 clove garlic, minced
- 2 tablespoons grated Parmesan cheese (optional)
- Salt and pepper to taste

Instructions:
1. Prepare the Croutons: Preheat your oven to 350°F (175°C). In a mixing bowl, toss the bread cubes with olive oil, garlic powder, oregano, salt, and pepper until evenly coated. Spread the cubes in a single layer on a baking sheet and bake for 10-12 minutes, or until golden and crispy. Set aside.
2. Prepare the Dressing: In a small bowl, whisk together the Greek yogurt, mayonnaise, lemon juice, Dijon mustard, minced garlic, Parmesan cheese, salt, and pepper until smooth and well combined. Adjust seasoning to taste.
3. Assemble the Salad: In a large salad bowl, combine the chopped romaine lettuce, sliced chicken breast, and cherry tomatoes if using. Add the homemade croutons and gently toss the salad with the dressing.
4. Serve: Divide the salad among four plates, sprinkle with additional Parmesan cheese if desired, and serve immediately.

Nutritional Information: *350 calories, 28g protein, 15g carbohydrates, 20g fats, 3g fiber, 85mg cholesterol, 350mg sodium, 700mg potassium.*

Sweet Potato, Cilantro, and Black Bean Salad
An energizing and hearty salad, perfect for lunch.

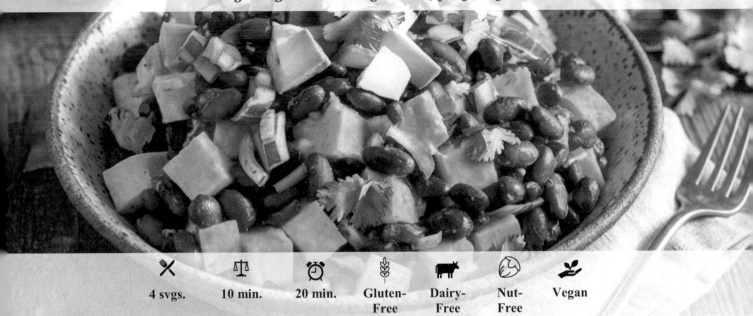

4 svgs.	10 min.	20 min.	Gluten-Free	Dairy-Free	Nut-Free	Vegan

Ingredients:

- 2 medium sweet potatoes, peeled and diced
- 1 can (15 oz) black beans, drained and rinsed
- 1/4 cup fresh cilantro, chopped
- 1/4 red onion, finely chopped
- 1 avocado, diced (optional)
- 2 tablespoons extra virgin olive oil
- 1 tablespoon lime juice
- 1 teaspoon ground cumin
- 1/2 teaspoon smoked paprika
- Salt and pepper to taste

Instructions:

1. Cook the Sweet Potatoes: In a large pot, bring water to a boil. Add the diced sweet potatoes and cook for about 10 minutes, or until tender but not mushy. Drain and let cool slightly.
2. Assemble the Salad: In a large mixing bowl, combine the cooked sweet potatoes, black beans, chopped cilantro, red onion, and diced avocado (if using).
3. Make the Dressing: In a small bowl, whisk together the olive oil, lime juice, ground cumin, smoked paprika, salt, and pepper until well combined.
4. Dress the Salad: Pour the dressing over the salad and toss gently to combine. Adjust seasoning to taste.
5. Serve: Serve the salad warm or at room temperature, and enjoy the vibrant flavors and nourishing ingredients.

Nutritional Information: *250 calories, 5g protein, 35g carbohydrates, 10g fats, 10g fiber, 0mg cholesterol, 200mg sodium, 600mg potassium.*

Notes:
Sweet potatoes are rich in beta-carotene and fiber, which support healthy digestion and reduce inflammation. **Black beans** add plant-based protein and additional fiber, making this salad a hearty and satisfying option for an anti-inflammatory diet. The **fresh cilantro** and lime juice add a burst of flavor, tying all the ingredients together beautifully.

Burrata, Basil, and Tomato Salad
A light and fresh salad, rich in calcium and antioxidants.

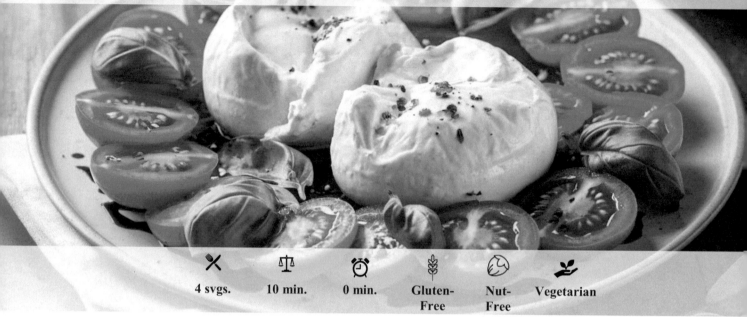

4 svgs.	10 min.	0 min.	Gluten-Free	Nut-Free	Vegetarian

Ingredients:
- 2 balls of fresh burrata cheese
- 2 cups cherry tomatoes, halved
- 1/4 cup fresh basil leaves, torn or chopped
- 2 tablespoons extra virgin olive oil
- 1 tablespoon balsamic glaze or balsamic vinegar
- Salt and pepper to taste
- Optional: A pinch of red pepper flakes for a touch of heat

Instructions:
1. Prepare the Tomatoes: In a large mixing bowl, combine the halved cherry tomatoes with a pinch of salt and pepper. Drizzle with 1 tablespoon of olive oil and toss gently to coat.
2. Assemble the Salad: Arrange the cherry tomatoes on a serving platter. Tear the burrata into pieces and place them evenly over the tomatoes. Scatter the fresh basil leaves on top.
3. Finish the Salad: Drizzle the salad with the remaining olive oil and balsamic glaze or vinegar. Add a pinch of red pepper flakes if desired.
4. Serve: Serve immediately, allowing the creaminess of the burrata to mingle with the juicy tomatoes and fragrant basil.

Nutritional Information: *280 calories, 10g protein, 7g carbohydrates, 24g fats, 2g fiber, 40mg cholesterol, 150mg sodium, 300mg potassium.*

Notes:
Burrata *is a rich source of calcium and healthy fats, while tomatoes provide lycopene, a powerful antioxidant that reduces inflammation. The combination of creamy burrata, sweet tomatoes, and fresh basil makes this salad a delicious and satisfying choice for an anti-inflammatory diet.*

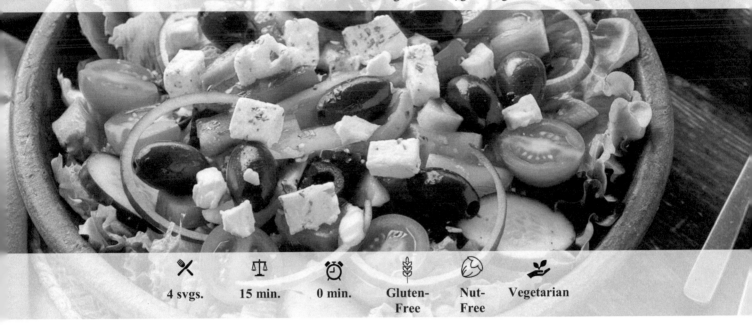

Greek Salad with Olives and Feta
A traditional salad with Mediterranean flavors, full of taste and goodness.

4 svgs.	15 min.	0 min.	Gluten-Free	Nut-Free	Vegetarian

Ingredients:

- 3 cups chopped romaine lettuce
- 1 cup cherry tomatoes, halved
- 1 cucumber, sliced into half-moons
- 1/2 red onion, thinly sliced
- 1/2 cup Kalamata olives, pitted and halved
- 1/4 cup green bell pepper, thinly sliced
- 4 oz feta cheese, crumbled or cubed
- 2 tablespoons extra virgin olive oil
- 1 tablespoon red wine vinegar
- 1 teaspoon dried oregano
- Salt and pepper to taste

Instructions:

1. Prepare the Vegetables: In a large salad bowl, combine the chopped romaine lettuce, cherry tomatoes, cucumber slices, red onion, Kalamata olives, and green bell pepper.
2. Add the Feta: Scatter the crumbled or cubed feta cheese over the salad.
3. Make the Dressing: In a small bowl, whisk together the olive oil, red wine vinegar, dried oregano, salt, and pepper until well combined.
4. Dress the Salad: Drizzle the dressing over the salad and toss gently to combine all the ingredients evenly.
5. Serve: Serve immediately, enjoying the crisp, fresh flavors and the savory richness of the feta cheese.

Nutritional Information: *220 calories, 7g protein, 10g carbohydrates, 18g fats, 4g fiber, 20mg cholesterol, 450mg sodium, 300mg potassium.*

Notes:
Greek salad is a classic dish rich in antioxidants and healthy fats. The combination of olives and olive oil provides heart-healthy monounsaturated fats, while the vegetables offer a variety of vitamins and minerals that help reduce inflammation. Feta cheese adds a tangy, creamy element, making this salad both flavorful and satisfying.

Niçoise Salad with Tuna and Egg
A nourishing salad with olive oil, olives, and fresh vegetables.

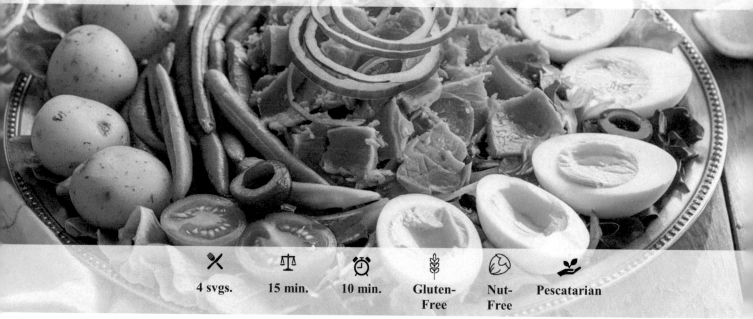

🍴 4 svgs.　⚖️ 15 min.　⏰ 10 min.　🌾 Gluten-Free　🌍 Nut-Free　🌱 Pescatarian

Ingredients:
- 2 cups baby potatoes, halved
- 2 cups green beans, trimmed
- 4 large eggs
- 1 can (5 oz) tuna in olive oil, drained
- 4 cups mixed greens (such as romaine, arugula, or spinach)
- 1/2 cup cherry tomatoes, halved
- 1/4 cup Kalamata olives, pitted
- 1/4 red onion, thinly sliced
- 1/4 cup fresh basil leaves, torn (optional)
- 2 tablespoons capers (optional)

For the Dressing:
- 1/4 cup extra virgin olive oil
- 1 tablespoon Dijon mustard
- 1 tablespoon red wine vinegar
- 1 teaspoon lemon juice
- 1 clove garlic, minced
- Salt and pepper to taste

Instructions:
1. Cook the Potatoes and Green Beans: Bring a pot of salted water to a boil. Add the baby potatoes and cook until tender, about 8-10 minutes. In the last 2 minutes of cooking, add the green beans. Drain and set aside to cool slightly.
2. Cook the Eggs: In a separate pot, bring water to a boil. Gently add the eggs and cook for 8-10 minutes for hard-boiled eggs. Transfer to an ice bath to cool, then peel and halve.
3. Assemble the Salad: On a large serving platter or individual plates, arrange the mixed greens. Top with the cooked potatoes, green beans, halved eggs, drained tuna, cherry tomatoes, Kalamata olives, red onion, basil leaves, and capers.
4. Make the Dressing: In a small bowl, whisk together the olive oil, Dijon mustard, red wine vinegar, lemon juice, minced garlic, salt, and pepper until well combined.
5. Dress the Salad: Drizzle the dressing over the salad and serve immediately.

Nutritional Information: *350 calories, 18g protein, 20g carbohydrates, 22g fats, 6g fiber, 200mg cholesterol, 350mg sodium, 700mg potassium.*

Notes:
Niçoise salad is a perfect combination of protein, healthy fats, and fiber, making it a well-rounded meal. Tuna provides omega-3 fatty acids, which have anti-inflammatory properties, while the variety of vegetables offers essential vitamins and minerals to support overall health.

Beet Salad with Goat Cheese and Pecans
Earthy notes of beetroot pair perfectly with creamy cheese and crunchy pecans.

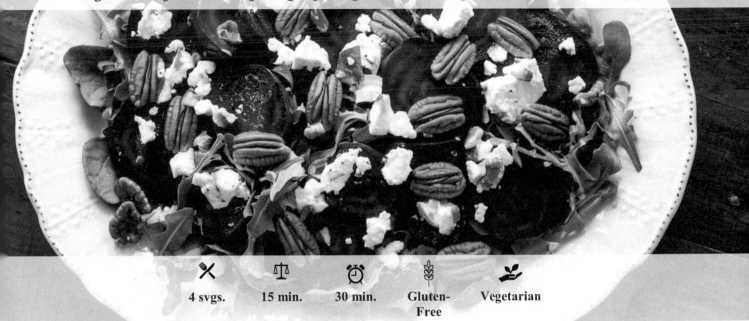

✕	⚖	⏰	🌾	🌱
4 svgs.	15 min.	30 min.	Gluten-Free	Vegetarian

Ingredients:
- 4 medium beets, roasted and sliced
- 4 oz goat cheese, crumbled
- 1/2 cup pecans, toasted and chopped
- 4 cups mixed greens (such as arugula or spinach)
- 1/4 red onion, thinly sliced
- 2 tablespoons extra virgin olive oil
- 1 tablespoon balsamic vinegar
- 1 teaspoon honey or maple syrup (optional)
- Salt and pepper to taste

Instructions:
1. Roast the Beets: Preheat your oven to 400°F (200°C). Wrap each beet in aluminum foil and roast on a baking sheet for about 30-40 minutes, or until tender. Allow the beets to cool, then peel and slice them into rounds.
2. Assemble the Salad: In a large salad bowl, combine the mixed greens, sliced beets, crumbled goat cheese, toasted pecans, and thinly sliced red onion.
3. Make the Dressing: In a small bowl, whisk together the olive oil, balsamic vinegar, honey or maple syrup (if using), salt, and pepper until well combined.
4. Dress the Salad: Drizzle the dressing over the salad and toss gently to combine. Adjust seasoning to taste.
5. Serve: Serve immediately, enjoying the rich flavors and creamy texture of this anti-inflammatory salad.

Nutritional Information: *300 calories, 8g protein, 22g carbohydrates, 22g fats, 6g fiber, 15mg cholesterol, 150mg sodium, 500mg potassium.*

Notes:
Beets *are rich in antioxidants and anti-inflammatory compounds like betalains, which give them their vibrant color. Paired with creamy goat cheese and crunchy pecans, this salad offers a delightful combination of textures and flavors, making it a perfect choice for a nutritious and satisfying meal.*

Artichoke, Pepper, and Arugula Salad
A salad with bold and vibrant flavors that will surprise and delight.

4 svgs. | 15 min. | 0 min. | Gluten-Free | Dairy-Free | Nut-Free | Vegan

Ingredients:
- 4 cups fresh arugula
- 1 can (14 oz) artichoke hearts, drained and quartered
- 1 red bell pepper, thinly sliced
- 1 yellow bell pepper, thinly sliced
- 1/4 cup red onion, thinly sliced
- 1/4 cup Kalamata olives, pitted and halved
- 2 tablespoons capers (optional)
- 3 tablespoons extra virgin olive oil
- 1 tablespoon lemon juice
- 1 teaspoon Dijon mustard
- Salt and pepper to taste

Instructions:
1. Prepare the Vegetables: In a large salad bowl, combine the fresh arugula, quartered artichoke hearts, sliced red and yellow bell peppers, sliced red onion, Kalamata olives, and capers if using.
2. Make the Dressing: In a small bowl, whisk together the olive oil, lemon juice, Dijon mustard, salt, and pepper until well combined.
3. Dress the Salad: Pour the dressing over the salad and toss gently to combine all the ingredients evenly.
4. Serve: Serve immediately, enjoying the crisp, fresh flavors and the savory richness of the artichokes and olives.

Nutritional Information: *180 calories, 3g protein, 12g carbohydrates, 14g fats, 4g fiber, 0mg cholesterol, 300mg sodium, 400mg potassium.*

Notes:
Artichokes *are a rich source of fiber and antioxidants, which help reduce inflammation and support digestive health. They are also packed with vitamins C and K, which boost immune function and promote healthy bones. Artichokes contain important minerals like magnesium, potassium, and phosphorus, which support heart health and muscle function. Additionally, they are a good source of folate, which is essential for cell growth and repair. Combined with the peppery flavor of arugula and the vibrant bell peppers, this salad is a flavorful and nutrient-dense choice for an anti-inflammatory diet.*

Kale and Pomegranate Salad with Tahini Dressing

An antioxidant-rich salad that combines crunchy textures and vibrant flavors

4 svgs.	15 min.	0 min.	Gluten-Free	Dairy-Free	Vegan

Ingredients:

- 4 cups kale, stems removed, leaves finely chopped
- 1/2 cup pomegranate seeds
- 1/4 cup sliced almonds, toasted
- 1 tbsp olive oil (for massaging the kale)

For the Lemon Tahini Dressing:

- 2 tbsp tahini
- 2 tbsp fresh lemon juice
- 1 tbsp olive oil
- 1 tsp maple syrup or honey
- 1 garlic clove, minced
- 1/4 tsp sea salt
- Freshly ground black pepper, to taste
- 2-3 tbsp water (to thin the dressing as needed)

Instructions:

1. Prepare the Kale: Place the chopped kale in a large bowl. Drizzle with 1 tbsp olive oil and massage the leaves with your hands for 2-3 minutes until they soften and darken in color.
2. Make the Dressing: In a small bowl, whisk together the tahini, lemon juice, olive oil, maple syrup (or honey), minced garlic, sea salt, and black pepper. Add water, one tablespoon at a time, until you reach a smooth, pourable consistency.
3. Assemble the Salad: Toss the massaged kale with the pomegranate seeds and toasted almonds.
4. Add the Dressing: Drizzle the lemon tahini dressing over the salad and toss gently to combine. Serve immediately.

Nutrition Information: 200 calories, 6g protein, 15g carbohydrates, 14g fat, 5g fiber, 0mg cholesterol, 120mg sodium, 300mg potassium

Notes:
Kale is a cruciferous vegetable loaded with vitamins A, C, and K, all of which have anti-inflammatory properties. Pomegranate seeds are rich in antioxidants, especially polyphenols, which help reduce inflammation and support heart health. Almonds add healthy fats and fiber, making this salad both delicious and nutritious

SOUPS: WARM AND RICH FLAVORS

Sweet Potato Soup with Ginger and Coconut Milk

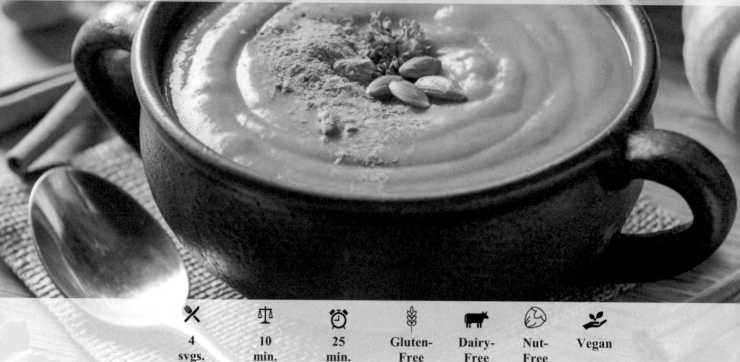

4 svgs.	10 min.	25 min.	Gluten-Free	Dairy-Free	Nut-Free	Vegan

Ingredients:

- 1 tablespoon coconut oil (or olive oil)
- 1 medium onion, chopped
- 2 cloves garlic, minced
- 1 tablespoon fresh ginger, grated
- 4 cups sweet potatoes, peeled and cubed
- 1 can (14 oz) coconut milk
- 1 teaspoon ground turmeric (optional)
- Salt and pepper to taste
- Fresh cilantro or green onions for garnish

Instructions:

1. Sauté the Aromatics: In a large pot, heat the coconut oil over medium heat. Add the chopped onion and sauté for about 5 minutes until softened. Add the minced garlic and grated ginger, and cook for another minute until fragrant.
2. Cook the Sweet Potatoes: Add the cubed sweet potatoes and vegetable broth to the pot. Bring to a boil, then reduce the heat and let it simmer for about 15-20 minutes, or until the sweet potatoes are tender.
3. Blend the Soup: Use an immersion blender to puree the soup until smooth, or transfer the soup in batches to a blender and blend until smooth. Return the soup to the pot if using a blender.
4. Add Coconut Milk: Stir in the coconut milk and ground turmeric (if using). Season with salt and pepper to taste. Reheat the soup gently, if needed, but do not let it boil.
5. Serve: Ladle the soup into bowls and garnish with fresh cilantro or green onions. Enjoy the rich, creamy texture and warming flavors of this anti-inflammatory soup.

Nutritional Information: 250 calories, 4g protein, 35g carbohydrates, 12g fats, 6g fiber, 0mg cholesterol, 350mg sodium, 700mg potassium.

Chicken Vegetable Soup with Thyme

A classic comforting soup, perfect for soothing the soul and supporting the immune system.

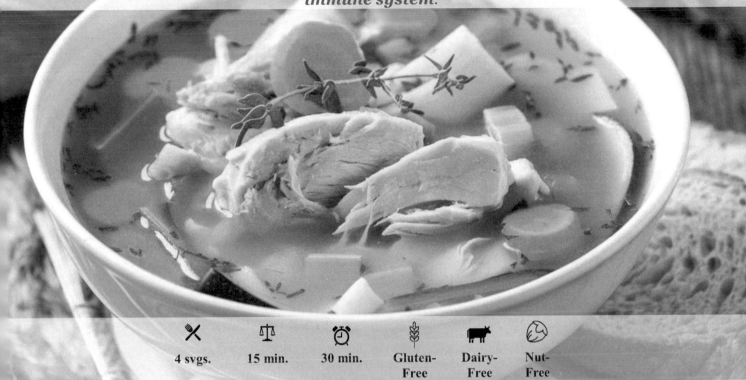

4 svgs.	15 min.	30 min.	Gluten-Free	Dairy-Free	Nut-Free

Ingredients:
- 1 tablespoon olive oil
- 1 medium onion, chopped
- 2 cloves garlic, minced
- 2 medium carrots, sliced
- 2 celery stalks, sliced
- 1 zucchini, diced
- 1 pound boneless, skinless chicken breasts, cut into bite-sized pieces
- 6 cups chicken broth
- 2 sprigs fresh thyme (or 1/2 teaspoon dried thyme)
- 1 bay leaf
- Salt and pepper to taste
- Fresh parsley for garnish

Instructions:
1. Sauté the Aromatics: In a large pot, heat the olive oil over medium heat. Add the chopped onion and sauté for about 5 minutes until softened. Add the minced garlic and cook for another minute until fragrant.
2. Cook the Chicken: Add the chicken pieces to the pot and cook until they are lightly browned on all sides, about 5 minutes.
3. Add Vegetables and Broth: Stir in the sliced carrots, celery, and zucchini. Pour in the chicken broth, then add the thyme sprigs and bay leaf. Bring the soup to a boil, then reduce the heat and let it simmer for about 20-25 minutes, or until the chicken is cooked through and the vegetables are tender.
4. Season and Serve: Remove the thyme sprigs and bay leaf. Season the soup with salt and pepper to taste. Ladle the soup into bowls and garnish with fresh parsley before serving.

Nutritional Information: *250 calories, 25g protein, 15g carbohydrates, 8g fats, 4g fiber, 60mg cholesterol, 700mg sodium, 800mg potassium.*

Creamy Broccoli Soup with Almond Milk

A smooth and creamy soup, rich in vitamin C and fiber.

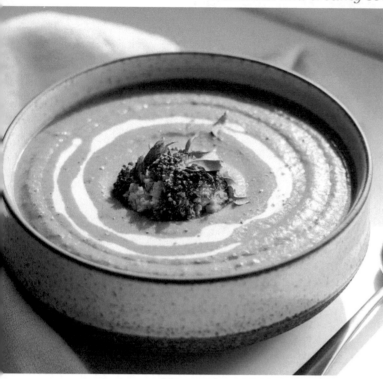

✗	⚖	⏱	🌾	🐄	🌱
4 svgs.	10 min.	20 min.	Gluten-Free	Dairy-Free	Vegan

Ingredients:

- 1 tablespoon olive oil
- 1 small onion, chopped
- 2 cloves garlic, minced
- 4 cups broccoli florets
- 4 cups vegetable broth
- 1 cup unsweetened almond milk (or oat milk for a nut-free version)
- 1/4 teaspoon ground nutmeg (optional)
- Salt and pepper to taste
- Fresh lemon juice to taste
- Fresh parsley or chives for garnish

Instructions:

1. Sauté the Aromatics: In a large pot, heat the olive oil over medium heat. Add the chopped onion and sauté for about 5 minutes until softened. Add the minced garlic and cook for another minute until fragrant.
2. Cook the Broccoli: Add the broccoli florets to the pot and pour in the vegetable broth. Bring to a boil, then reduce the heat and simmer for about 10-15 minutes, until the broccoli is tender.
3. Blend the Soup: Use an immersion blender to puree the soup until smooth, or transfer the soup in batches to a blender and blend until smooth. Return the soup to the pot if using a blender.
4. Add Almond Milk: Stir in the almond milk and ground nutmeg, if using. Season with salt, pepper, and a squeeze of fresh lemon juice to taste. Reheat the soup gently, if needed, but do not let it boil.
5. Serve: Ladle the soup into bowls, garnish with fresh parsley or chives, and enjoy this creamy, anti-inflammatory soup.

Nutritional Information: 150 calories, 4g protein, 15g carbohydrates, 8g fats, 4g fiber, 0mg cholesterol, 300mg sodium, 500mg potassium.

Notes:
Broccoli *is packed with vitamins C and K, as well as powerful antioxidants that help reduce inflammation. Almond milk adds a creamy texture without dairy, making this soup both nutritious and gentle on the digestive system. This soothing soup is perfect for a light lunch or a comforting dinner.*

Tomato Soup with Basil and Garlic
A fragrant soup rich in antioxidants that help combat inflammation

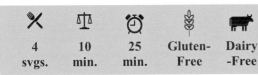						
4 svgs.	10 min.	25 min.	Gluten-Free	Dairy-Free	Nut-Free	Vegan

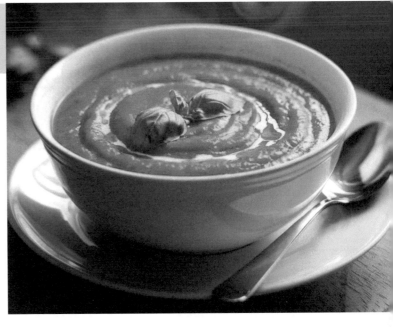

Ingredients:
- 1 tablespoon olive oil
- 1 medium onion, chopped
- 4 cloves garlic, minced
- 6 cups ripe tomatoes, chopped (or two 28 oz cans of crushed tomatoes)
- 2 cups vegetable broth
- 1/2 cup fresh basil leaves, chopped
- 1 tablespoon tomato paste
- 1 teaspoon balsamic vinegar
- Salt and pepper to taste
- Fresh basil leaves for garnish

Instructions:
1. Sauté the Aromatics: Heat the olive oil over medium heat in a large pot. Add the chopped onion and sauté for about 5 minutes until softened. Add the minced garlic and cook for another minute until fragrant.
2. Cook the Tomatoes: Add the chopped tomatoes (or crushed tomatoes) and tomato paste to the pot. Pour in the vegetable broth and bring to a boil. Reduce the heat and let the soup simmer for about 20 minutes, allowing the flavors to meld together.
3. Blend the Soup: Use an immersion blender to puree the soup until smooth, or transfer the soup in batches to a blender and blend until smooth. Return the soup to the pot if using a blender.
4. Add Basil and Season: Stir in the chopped basil, balsamic vinegar, salt, and pepper. Taste and adjust the seasoning as needed. Reheat gently if necessary.
5. Serve: Ladle the soup into bowls and garnish with fresh basil leaves. Enjoy this rich, flavorful anti-inflammatory soup.

Nutritional Information: 180 calories, 4g protein, 22g carbohydrates, 8g fats, 5g fiber, 0mg cholesterol, 350mg sodium, 700mg potassium.

Notes:
Tomatoes *are rich in lycopene, a powerful antioxidant known for its anti-inflammatory properties. Paired with fresh basil and garlic, this soup not only offers robust flavor but also provides health benefits that support a balanced, anti-inflammatory diet. Perfect as a starter or a light meal on its own*

Lentil Soup with Turmeric and Spinach

A nourishing soup that boosts immunity and supports heart health.

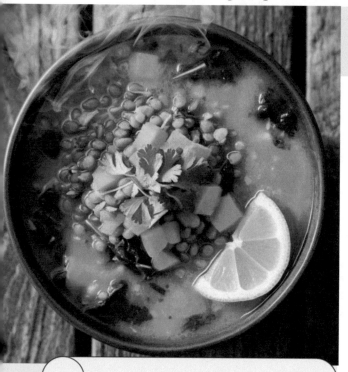

✗	⚖	⏰	Gluten-Free	Dairy-Free	Nut-Free	Vegan
4 svgs.	10 min.	30 min.				

Ingredients:

- 1 tablespoon olive oil
- 1 medium onion, chopped
- 2 cloves garlic, minced
- 1 teaspoon ground turmeric
- 1 teaspoon ground cumin
- 1 cup dried lentils, rinsed
- 4 cups vegetable broth (or chicken broth for non-vegan)
- 2 cups water
- 2 cups fresh spinach leaves
- 1 medium carrot, diced
- 1 celery stalk, diced
- 1 bay leaf
- Salt and pepper to taste
- Fresh lemon juice to taste
- Fresh cilantro or parsley for garnish

Instructions:

1. Sauté the Aromatics: In a large pot, heat the olive oil over medium heat. Add the chopped onion and sauté for about 5 minutes until softened. Add the minced garlic, ground turmeric, and ground cumin, and cook for another minute until fragrant.
2. Cook the Lentils: Add the rinsed lentils, diced carrot, diced celery, vegetable broth, water, and bay leaf to the pot. Bring to a boil, then reduce the heat and simmer for about 25 minutes, or until the lentils are tender.
3. Add the Spinach: Stir in the fresh spinach leaves and cook for an additional 2-3 minutes until wilted. Remove the bay leaf, then season the soup with salt, pepper, and a squeeze of fresh lemon juice to taste.
4. Serve: Ladle the soup into bowls and garnish with fresh cilantro or parsley. Enjoy this hearty, anti-inflammatory soup.

Nutritional Information: *220 calories, 12g protein, 32g carbohydrates, 5g fats, 12g fiber, 0mg cholesterol, 300mg sodium, 700mg potassium.*

Notes:

Lentils *are an excellent source of plant-based protein and fiber, which help reduce inflammation and support digestive health. They are also rich in essential vitamins and minerals, including iron, which supports oxygen transport in the blood, and folate, which is crucial for DNA synthesis and cell growth. Lentils provide a good amount of magnesium, potassium, and zinc, which are important for heart health, immune function, and maintaining healthy skin. They are also high in B vitamins like B1 (thiamine), B6, and B9 (folate), which play a key role in energy metabolism and nervous system health.*

Turmeric, *known for its active compound curcumin, has powerful anti-inflammatory and antioxidant effects, helping to combat chronic inflammation and protect the body from oxidative damage.*

Seafood Broth with Fennel and Celery

A nutrient-rich soup, packed with omega-3s and minerals, that helps reduce inflammation.

✖	⚖	⏰	🌾	🐄	🌍	🌱
4 svgs.	15 min.	30 min.	Gluten -Free	Dairy -Free	Nut- Free	Pescat arian

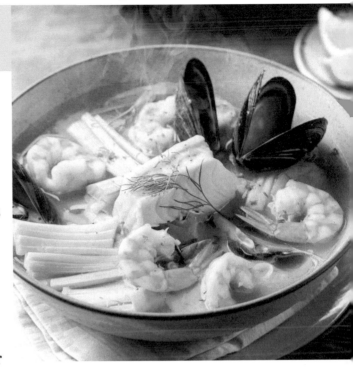

Ingredients:

- 1 tablespoon olive oil
- 1 small fennel bulb, thinly sliced
- 2 celery stalks, sliced
- 1 small onion, chopped
- 2 cloves garlic, minced
- 1/2 teaspoon crushed red pepper flakes (optional)
- 4 cups seafood or fish stock
- 1 cup dry white wine (optional)
- 1 bay leaf
- 1/2-pound mussels, cleaned
- 1/2-pound shrimp, peeled and deveined
- 1/2-pound firm white fish (such as cod or halibut), cut into bite-sized pieces
- Salt and pepper to taste
- Fresh parsley or dill for garnish
- Lemon wedges for serving

Instructions:

1. Sauté the Aromatics: In a large pot, heat the olive oil over medium heat. Add the sliced fennel, celery, and chopped onion, and sauté for about 5 minutes until softened. Add the minced garlic and crushed red pepper flakes (if using), and cook for another minute until fragrant.
2. Add the Broth: Pour in the seafood or fish stock and white wine (if using). Add the bay leaf and bring the mixture to a boil. Reduce the heat and let it simmer for about 10 minutes, allowing the flavors to meld together.
3. Cook the Seafood: Add the mussels, shrimp, and white fish to the pot. Cover and cook for about 5-7 minutes, or until the seafood is cooked through and the mussels have opened. Discard any mussels that do not open.
4. Season and Serve: Remove the bay leaf and season the broth with salt and pepper to taste. Ladle the seafood broth into bowls and garnish with fresh parsley or dill. Serve with lemon wedges on the side.

Nutritional Information: 250 calories, 25g protein, 8g carbohydrates, 10g fats, 2g fiber, 150mg cholesterol, 600mg sodium, 900mg potassium.

Notes:
Seafood *is rich in omega-3 fatty acids, which have powerful anti-inflammatory properties. Fennel and celery add a refreshing crunch and are known for their digestive benefits. This light yet flavorful broth is perfect for a nourishing, anti-inflammatory meal that feels both comforting and elegant.*

Miso Soup with Tofu and Seaweed
A Japanese soup that helps maintain a healthy balance of gut bacteria.

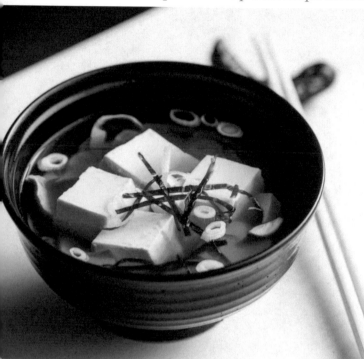

🍴	⚖️	⏰	🌾	🐄	🌍	🌱
4 svgs.	**10 min.**	**15 min.**	**Gluten-Free**	**Dairy-Free**	**Nut-Free**	**Vegan**

Ingredients:

- 4 cups water
- 1/4 cup miso paste (white or yellow)
- 1 cup firm tofu, cubed
- 1/4 cup dried wakame seaweed
- 2 green onions, sliced
- 1/2 cup sliced mushrooms (optional)
- 1 tablespoon soy sauce or tamari (optional for extra flavor)
- 1 tablespoon sesame oil (optional for drizzling)
- Freshly chopped green onions or cilantro for garnish

Instructions:

1. Prepare the Base: In a medium pot, bring the water to a gentle simmer. Add the sliced mushrooms (if using) and simmer for 5 minutes until tender.
2. Add the Miso: In a small bowl, mix the miso paste with a few tablespoons of hot water to dissolve it. Stir the dissolved miso into the pot. Reduce the heat to low to prevent boiling, as boiling can destroy the beneficial probiotics in miso.
3. Add Tofu and Seaweed: Add the cubed tofu and dried wakame seaweed to the pot. Let the seaweed rehydrate and the tofu warm through, about 2-3 minutes.
4. Finish the Soup: Stir in the soy sauce or tamari if using, and drizzle with sesame oil for added flavor. Taste and adjust seasoning as needed.
5. Serve: Ladle the miso soup into bowls and garnish with freshly sliced green onions or cilantro. Enjoy the savory, nourishing flavors of this traditional Japanese soup.

Nutritional Information: *100 calories, 7g protein, 6g carbohydrates, 6g fats, 1g fiber, 0mg cholesterol, 500mg sodium, 200mg potassium.*

Notes:
• **Miso** is a fermented soybean paste rich in probiotics, which support gut health and possess anti-inflammatory properties. It is also a good source of vitamins and minerals, including **vitamin K, manganese, and zinc**, which contribute to bone health, immune function, and wound healing. Combined with protein-rich tofu, which provides essential amino acids, and mineral-packed seaweed, rich in **iodine, calcium, and magnesium**, this miso soup is not only delicious but also highly nourishing. It's a perfect addition to an anti-inflammatory diet, supporting overall health and well-being.

Mushroom, Thyme, and Garlic Soup

A hearty, flavorful soup that boosts immunity and delivers a healthy dose of antioxidants.

✖	⚖	⏰	🌾	🐄	🌍	🌱
4 svgs.	**10 min.**	**25 min.**	**Gluten -Free**	**Dairy -Free**	**Nut- Free**	**Vegan**

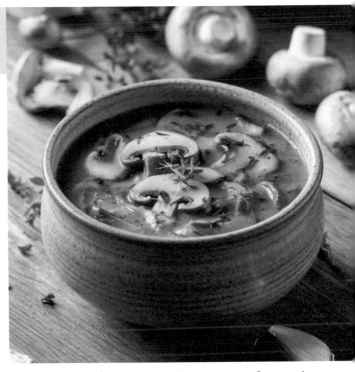

Ingredients:

- 1 lb mixed mushrooms (such as cremini, shiitake, and button), sliced
- 1 large onion, chopped
- 4 cloves garlic, minced
- 4 cups vegetable broth
- 1 tbsp fresh thyme leaves (or 1 tsp dried thyme)
- 2 tbsp olive oil
- 1/2 tsp sea salt
- 1/4 tsp freshly ground black pepper
- 1/4 cup chopped fresh parsley for garnish (optional)

Instructions:

1. In a large pot, heat the olive oil over medium heat. Add the chopped onion and sauté until softened, about 5 minutes.
2. Add the garlic and sliced mushrooms to the pot. Cook, stirring occasionally, until the mushrooms are browned and have released their moisture, about 8 minutes.
3. Stir in the thyme, salt, and pepper. Pour in the vegetable broth and bring the mixture to a boil. Reduce heat and let simmer for 15 minutes, allowing the flavors to meld together.
4. Serve hot, garnished with fresh parsley if desired.

Nutritional Information: *120 calories, 3g protein, 10g carbohydrates, 8g fat, 2g fiber, 0mg cholesterol, 400mg sodium, 450mg potassium*

Notes:

Mushrooms *are a fantastic source of vitamins and minerals, including B vitamins (such as B2 and B3), which support energy metabolism and brain function. They are also rich in selenium, a powerful antioxidant that helps reduce inflammation and protect cells from damage.*

Thyme *is not only a flavorful herb but also packed with vitamin C and vitamin A, both of which boost immune function and promote healthy skin.*

Garlic *is well-known for its anti-inflammatory and immune-boosting properties, thanks to its active compound, allicin, which helps reduce oxidative stress and supports cardiovascular health.*

Together, these ingredients make this soup both comforting and nutrient-dense, making it an ideal choice for a healthy, anti-inflammatory diet.

Rosemary and Lemon Baked Chicken Breast
A light and flavorful dish, perfect for supporting heart health.

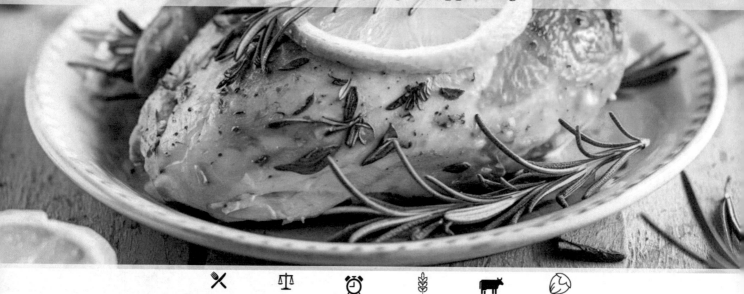

4 svgs.	**10** min.	**30** min.	Gluten-Free	Dairy-Free	Nut-Free

Ingredients:
- 4 boneless, skinless chicken breasts
- 2 lemons, thinly sliced
- 4 sprigs fresh rosemary
- 3 cloves garlic, minced
- 2 tbsp olive oil
- 1/2 tsp sea salt
- 1/4 tsp freshly ground black pepper

Instructions:
1. Preheat your oven to 375°F (190°C). Place the chicken breasts in a baking dish.
2. Drizzle the olive oil over the chicken, then sprinkle with minced garlic, sea salt, and black pepper.
3. Lay the lemon slices and rosemary sprigs over the chicken breasts.
4. Bake in the preheated oven for 25-30 minutes, or until the chicken is cooked through and reaches an internal temperature of 165°F (75°C).
5. Remove from the oven and let rest for a few minutes before serving. Garnish with additional lemon slices or rosemary if desired.

Nutrition Information: *220 calories, 28g protein, 2g carbohydrates, 10g fat, 0g fiber, 80mg cholesterol, 360mg sodium, 450mg potassium*

Notes:
Rosemary and Lemon Baked Chicken Breast *is a healthy, flavorful option packed with nutrients.* **Chicken breast** *is a lean source of high-quality protein, which supports muscle repair and overall health. It's also low in fat, making it heart-friendly.*
Rosemary *contains antioxidants and anti-inflammatory compounds that support the immune system and improve digestion. It's also rich in* **carnosic acid**, *which is believed to promote brain health.* **Lemon** *adds a dose of* **vitamin C**, *an important antioxidant that boosts the immune system, aids in collagen production, and enhances iron absorption.*

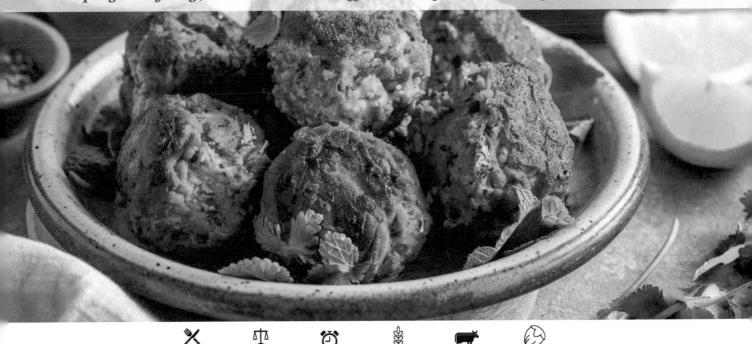

Turkish Meatballs with Cilantro and Mint
Spicy and juicy, these meatballs offer a rich flavor and digestive benefits.

| 4 svgs. | 15 min. | 20 min. | Gluten-Free | Dairy-Free | Nut-Free |

Ingredients:
- 1 lb ground beef
- 1/2 cup fresh cilantro, finely chopped
- 1/4 cup fresh mint, finely chopped
- 1 small onion, finely chopped
- 3 cloves garlic, minced
- 1 tsp ground cumin
- 1 tsp ground coriander
- 1/2 tsp sea salt
- 1/4 tsp freshly ground black pepper
- 1 tbsp olive oil (for frying)

Instructions:
1. In a large bowl, combine the ground meat, cilantro, mint, onion, garlic, cumin, coriander, salt, and pepper. Mix thoroughly until all ingredients are evenly distributed.
2. Shape the mixture into small meatballs, about the size of a walnut.
3. Heat olive oil in a large skillet over medium heat. Add the meatballs and cook, turning occasionally, until browned on all sides and cooked through, about 15-20 minutes.
4. Serve hot, garnished with additional fresh cilantro or mint if desired. These meatballs pair well with a side of yogurt sauce or fresh salad.

Nutrition Information: 250 calories, 20g protein, 3g carbohydrates, 18g fat, 1g fiber, 70mg cholesterol, 350mg sodium, 400mg potassium

Notes:
Ground meat *provides a good source of protein, essential for muscle repair and overall body function.* **Cilantro** *is known for its digestive benefits and detoxifying properties, helping to eliminate heavy metals from the body. It's also rich in* **vitamin K**, *which supports bone health.* **Mint** *is refreshing and soothing, aiding digestion and helping to relieve indigestion or bloating. It also contains* **antioxidants** *and* **anti-inflammatory compounds** *that promote respiratory health.*

Duck with Orange Sauce and Thyme

This dish combines rich flavors and healthy fats, helping to reduce inflammation.

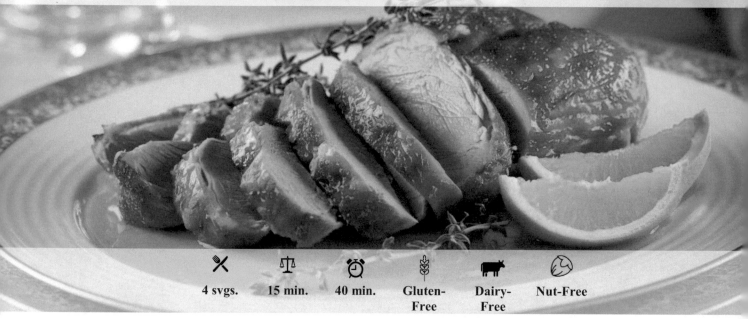

| 4 svgs. | 15 min. | 40 min. | Gluten-Free | Dairy-Free | Nut-Free |

Ingredients:

- 2 duck breasts, skin-on
- 1 cup freshly squeezed orange juice (about 2-3 oranges)
- Zest of 1 orange
- 1/4 cup honey
- 1 tbsp balsamic vinegar
- 2 sprigs fresh thyme
- 2 cloves garlic, minced
- 1/2 tsp sea salt
- 1/4 tsp freshly ground black pepper

Instructions:

1. Preheat your oven to 400°F (200°C). Score the skin of the duck breasts in a crisscross pattern, being careful not to cut into the meat. Season both sides with sea salt and black pepper.
2. Heat a large oven-safe skillet over medium heat. Place the duck breasts skin-side down and cook until the skin is crispy and golden, about 6-8 minutes. Flip the breasts and sear the other side for 2 minutes.
3. Transfer the skillet to the preheated oven and roast for 10-12 minutes for medium-rare, or until the internal temperature reaches 135°F (57°C). Remove from the oven and let the duck rest while you prepare the sauce.
4. In a small saucepan, combine orange juice, orange zest, honey, balsamic vinegar, thyme sprigs, and minced garlic. Bring to a boil, then reduce heat and simmer until the sauce thickens, about 10 minutes. Remove thyme sprigs.
5. Slice the duck breasts and drizzle with the orange sauce. Serve immediately.

Nutrition Information: *350 calories, 30g protein, 15g carbohydrates, 20g fat, 0g fiber, 120mg cholesterol, 320mg sodium, 400mg potassium.*

> **Notes:**
> ***The oranges*** *are rich in vitamin C, which acts as a powerful antioxidant, helping to reduce inflammation and boost the immune system?*
> ***Thyme*** *also contributes with its anti-inflammatory and antimicrobial properties, making this dish not only flavorful but also beneficial for your health.*

Honey Mustard Chicken Wings

A touch of sweetness and spice for a delightful treat without compromising your health.

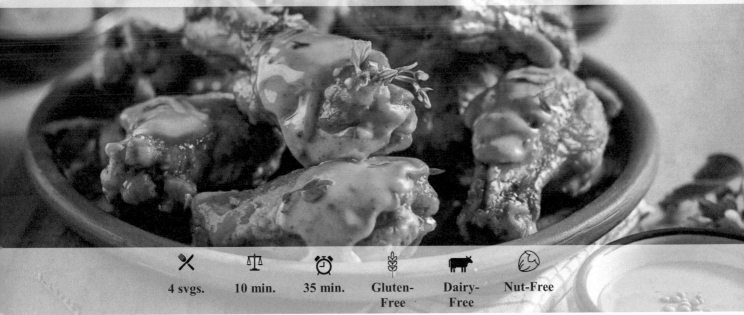

4 svgs.	10 min.	35 min.	Gluten-Free	Dairy-Free	Nut-Free

Ingredients:

- 2 lbs chicken wings
- 1/4 cup honey
- 2 tbsp Dijon mustard
- 2 tbsp whole grain mustard
- 1 tbsp apple cider vinegar
- 2 cloves garlic, minced
- 1 tsp paprika
- 1/2 tsp sea salt
- 1/4 tsp freshly ground black pepper
- 1 tbsp olive oil

Instructions:

1. Preheat your oven to 400°F (200°C). Line a baking sheet with parchment paper or lightly grease it.
2. In a large bowl, whisk together the honey, Dijon mustard, whole grain mustard, apple cider vinegar, garlic, paprika, salt, and pepper. Add the chicken wings to the bowl and toss until they are evenly coated in the sauce.
3. Place the wings in a single layer on the prepared baking sheet. Bake in the preheated oven for 30-35 minutes, or until the wings are golden and crispy, flipping halfway through cooking.
4. Serve the wings hot, garnished with fresh herbs if desired.

Nutrition Information:320 calories, 20g protein, 15g carbohydrates, 20g fat, 0g fiber, 100mg cholesterol, 420mg sodium, 300mg potassium

Notes:
Chicken wings *provide a good source of protein, essential for tissue repair and maintaining muscle mass.*
Honey *in this dish not only adds natural sweetness but is also rich in antioxidants, which support the immune system and reduce inflammation. It also has antibacterial properties.*
Mustard *aids digestion and contains* **selenium**, *which supports heart health and offers antioxidant benefits. Its spicy components can also help boost metabolism.*

Turkey with Cranberry Sauce and Quinoa

A festive dish with a sweet and tangy flavor is rich in antioxidants.

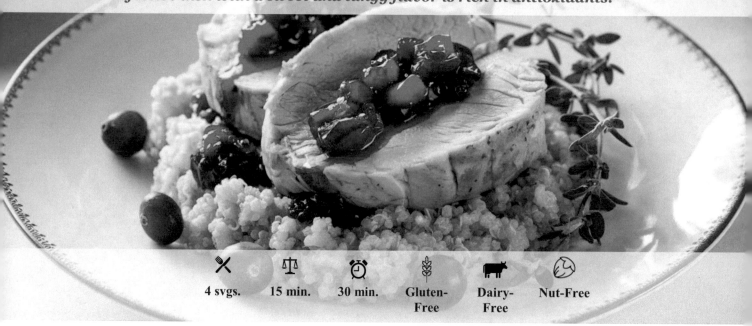

| 4 svgs. | 15 min. | 30 min. | Gluten-Free | Dairy-Free | Nut-Free |

Ingredients:

- 1 lb turkey breast, sliced into medallions
- 1 cup quinoa, rinsed
- 2 cups water or chicken broth
- 1 cup fresh or frozen cranberries
- 1/4 cup honey or maple syrup
- 1/4 cup orange juice
- 1 tbsp olive oil
- 1 tsp fresh thyme leaves (or 1/2 tsp dried thyme)
- 1/2 tsp sea salt
- 1/4 tsp freshly ground black pepper

Instructions:

1. In a medium saucepan, bring the water or chicken broth to a boil. Add the quinoa, reduce the heat to low, cover, and simmer for about 15 minutes, or until the quinoa is cooked and the liquid is absorbed. Fluff with a fork and set aside.
2. In a small saucepan, combine the cranberries, honey or maple syrup, and orange juice. Cook over medium heat until the cranberries burst and the sauce thickens, about 10 minutes. Set aside.
3. While the quinoa and sauce are cooking, heat the olive oil in a large skillet over medium-high heat. Season the turkey medallions with sea salt, black pepper, and thyme. Cook the turkey in the skillet for about 4-5 minutes per side, until golden brown and cooked through.
4. Serve the turkey medallions over the quinoa, drizzling the cranberry sauce on top. Garnish with additional thyme if desired.

Nutrition Information: *320 calories, 30g protein, 35g carbohydrates, 8g fat, 4g fiber, 70mg cholesterol, 350mg sodium, 500mg potassium*

Notes:

The cranberries *are rich in antioxidants, which help reduce inflammation and support urinary tract health.* **Quinoa** *is a complete protein, containing all nine essential amino acids, and is also high in fiber, making this dish both nourishing and beneficial for your health.*

Asian-Style Chicken with Ginger and Soy Sauce
Bold flavors that support the immune system and boost metabolism.

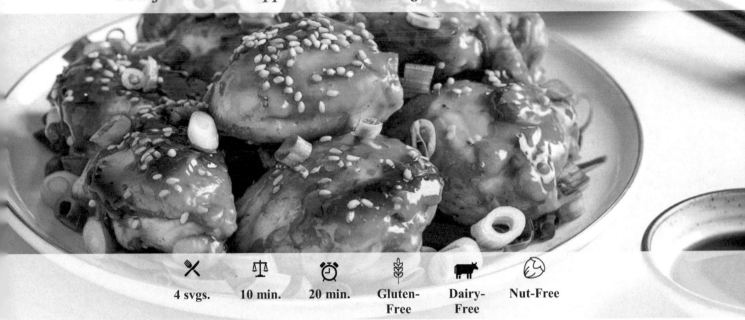

4 svgs.	10 min.	20 min.	Gluten-Free	Dairy-Free	Nut-Free

Ingredients:
- 1 lb boneless, skinless chicken thighs, cut into bite-sized pieces
- 2 tbsp gluten-free soy sauce (or tamari)
- 1 tbsp fresh ginger, minced
- 2 cloves garlic, minced
- 1 tbsp honey or maple syrup
- 1 tbsp rice vinegar
- 1 tbsp sesame oil
- 1/4 cup green onions, sliced
- 1/2 tsp red pepper flakes (optional, for a spicy kick)
- 1 tbsp sesame seeds (optional, for garnish)
- 2 tbsp vegetable oil

Instructions:
1. In a small bowl, mix together the soy sauce, honey, rice vinegar, sesame oil, ginger, and garlic. Set aside.
2. Heat the vegetable oil in a large skillet over medium-high heat. Add the chicken pieces and cook until browned and cooked through, about 8-10 minutes.
3. Pour the ginger-soy sauce mixture over the chicken in the skillet. Cook, stirring frequently, until the sauce thickens and coats the chicken, about 5 minutes.
4. Garnish with sliced green onions, sesame seeds, and red pepper flakes if using. Serve hot with steamed rice or your favorite vegetables.

Nutrition Information:
280 calories, 25g protein, 8g carbohydrates, 15g fat, 1g fiber, 90mg cholesterol, 750mg sodium, 350mg potassium

Notes:
The ginger is well-known for its anti-inflammatory and antioxidant properties. It helps reduce muscle pain and soreness, while also supporting digestion. **Soy sauce**, when used in moderation, provides a rich umami flavor and is low in calories, making this dish both flavorful and beneficial for your health.

Spinach and Feta Stuffed Turkey Breast
A healthy and delicious dish, perfect for lunch or dinner.

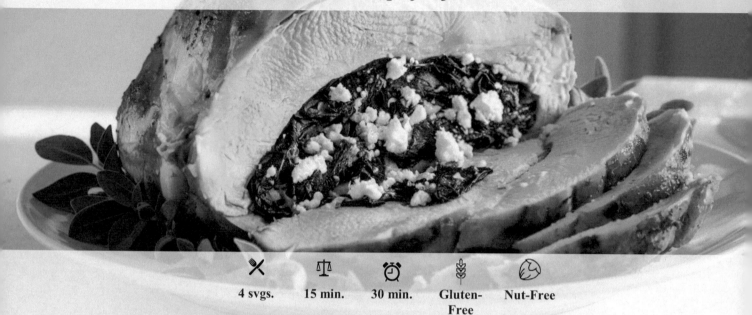

4 svgs. | **15 min.** | **30 min.** | **Gluten-Free** | **Nut-Free**

Ingredients:
- 1 lb turkey breast, butterflied and pounded thin
- 1 cup fresh spinach, chopped
- 1/2 cup crumbled feta cheese
- 2 cloves garlic, minced
- 1 tbsp olive oil
- 1 tsp fresh oregano, chopped (or 1/2 tsp dried oregano)
- 1/2 tsp sea salt
- 1/4 tsp freshly ground black pepper
- Toothpicks or kitchen twine for securing

Instructions:
1. Preheat your oven to 375°F (190°C). In a skillet, heat the olive oil over medium heat. Add the garlic and cook until fragrant, about 1 minute. Add the chopped spinach and cook until wilted, about 2-3 minutes. Remove from heat and let cool slightly.
2. In a bowl, combine the cooked spinach, crumbled feta, oregano, sea salt, and black pepper. Mix well.
3. Lay the butterflied turkey breast flat on a cutting board. Spread the spinach and feta mixture evenly over the surface of the turkey. Roll the turkey breast tightly, starting from one end, and secure with toothpicks or kitchen twine.
4. Place the stuffed turkey breast in a baking dish and bake in the preheated oven for 25-30 minutes, or until the internal temperature reaches 165°F (75°C).
5. Let the turkey rest for a few minutes before slicing and serving.

Nutrition Information: *320 calories, 35g protein, 10g carbohydrates, 15g fat, 2g fiber, 90mg cholesterol, 500mg sodium, 600mg potassium.*

Notes:
The spinach is a powerhouse of nutrients, rich in vitamins A, C, and K, as well as antioxidants that help reduce inflammation. **Feta cheese** adds a tangy flavor and provides calcium and protein, making this dish not only delicious but also beneficial for bone health and overall well-being.

Chicken Marsala with Mushrooms

A rich and elegant dish, perfect for a festive meal with tender chicken and savory mushrooms in a Marsala wine sauce.

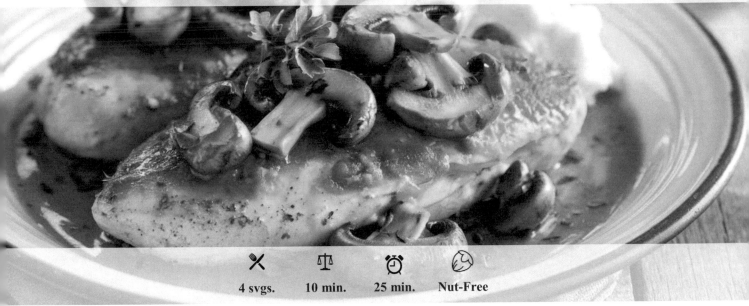

🍴 4 svgs.   ⚖ 10 min.   ⏰ 25 min.   🌐 Nut-Free

Ingredients:

- 4 boneless, skinless chicken breasts
- 1/2 cup all-purpose flour (or gluten-free alternative)
- 2 tablespoons olive oil
- 1 tablespoon butter
- 8 oz mushrooms, sliced
- 1/2 cup Marsala wine
- 1/2 cup chicken broth
- 1/4 cup heavy cream (optional)
- 2 cloves garlic, minced
- 1 teaspoon dried thyme (or 1 tablespoon fresh)
- Salt and pepper to taste
- Fresh parsley, chopped (for garnish)

Instructions:

1. Prepare the Chicken: Pound the chicken breasts to an even thickness. Season both sides with salt and pepper, then dredge in flour, shaking off the excess.
2. Cook the Chicken: Heat olive oil and butter in a large skillet over medium heat. Cook the chicken breasts for about 4-5 minutes per side, or until golden brown and cooked through. Remove the chicken from the skillet and set aside.
3. Cook the Mushrooms: In the same skillet, add the sliced mushrooms and sauté for 5-7 minutes, until browned. Add the minced garlic and thyme, cooking for another minute until fragrant.
4. Make the Sauce: Pour in the Marsala wine and chicken broth, scraping up any browned bits from the bottom of the skillet. Simmer the sauce for 5 minutes until it slightly reduces. For a richer sauce, stir in the heavy cream and cook for another 2-3 minutes.
5. Combine and Serve: Return the cooked chicken to the skillet, spooning the sauce and mushrooms over the top. Cook for an additional 2 minutes to warm the chicken through. Garnish with fresh parsley and serve with mashed potatoes, pasta, or vegetables.

Nutrition Information: *350 calories, 30g protein, 10g carbohydrates, 20g fats, 2g fiber, 80mg cholesterol, 400mg sodium, 500mg potassium.*

SEAFOOD AND FISH DISHES: *Fresh From The Sea*

Avocado and Salmon Salad
An excellent source of omega-3 fatty acids and healthy fats.

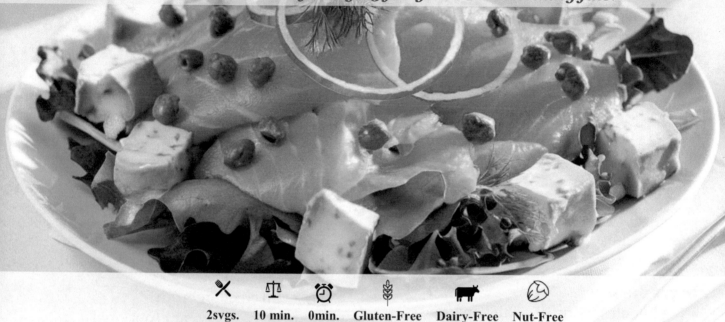

✗	⚖	⏰	🌾	🐄	🌍
2svgs.	10 min.	0min.	Gluten-Free	Dairy-Free	Nut-Free

Ingredients:

- 4 oz smoked salmon, thinly sliced
- 1 large avocado, peeled, pitted, and diced
- 1 cup mixed greens (such as arugula, spinach, or kale)
- 1/4 red onion, thinly sliced
- 1 tbsp capers (optional)

- 2 tbsp extra virgin olive oil
- 1 tbsp lemon juice
- 1 tsp Dijon mustard
- 1/2 tsp sea salt
- 1/4 tsp freshly ground black pepper
- Fresh dill for garnish (optional)

Instructions:

1. In a small bowl, whisk together the olive oil, lemon juice, Dijon mustard, sea salt, and black pepper to make the dressing.
2. In a large bowl, combine the mixed greens, avocado, red onion, and capers if using. Toss gently to mix.
3. Add the smoked salmon slices on top of the salad, then drizzle with the prepared dressing.
4. Garnish with fresh dill if desired and serve immediately.

Nutrition Information: 350 calories, 18g protein, 10g carbohydrates, 28g fat, 7g fiber, 35mg cholesterol, 600mg sodium, 900mg potassium.

Notes:
Avocados are rich in healthy monounsaturated fats that help reduce inflammation and support heart health. **Salmon** is an excellent source of omega-3 fatty acids, known for their powerful anti-inflammatory properties and benefits for both brain and cardiovascular health. This salad combines these two superfoods into a delicious and nutritious meal.

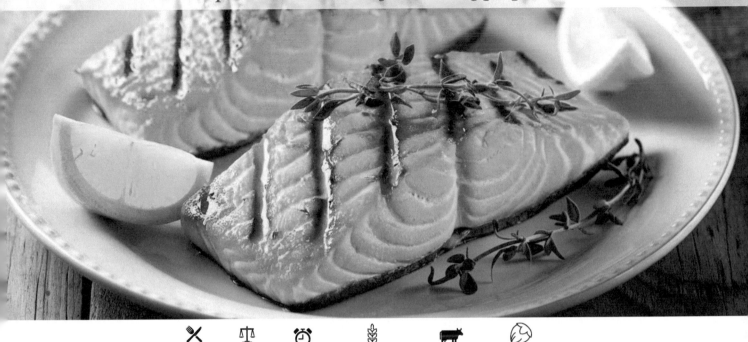

Grilled Salmon with Lemon-Thyme Marinade
A simple dish with anti-inflammatory properties

4 svgs.   10 min.   15 min.   Gluten-Free   Dairy-Free   Nut-Free

Ingredients:
- 4 salmon fillets (about 6 oz each)
- 2 tbsp fresh lemon juice
- 1 tbsp lemon zest
- 2 tbsp olive oil
- 2 cloves garlic, minced
- 2 tsp fresh thyme leaves (or 1 tsp dried thyme)
- 1/2 tsp sea salt
- 1/4 tsp freshly ground black pepper
- Lemon wedges for serving (optional)

Instructions:
1. In a small bowl, whisk together the lemon juice, lemon zest, olive oil, minced garlic, thyme, sea salt, and black pepper to make the marinade.
2. Place the salmon fillets in a shallow dish or a resealable plastic bag, and pour the marinade over them. Let the salmon marinate in the refrigerator for at least 30 minutes, or up to 2 hours.
3. Preheat your grill to medium-high heat. Remove the salmon from the marinade and grill skin-side down for about 6-8 minutes per side, or until the salmon is cooked through and has nice grill marks.
4. Serve the grilled salmon hot, garnished with lemon wedges if desired.

Nutrition Information: *350 calories, 30g protein, 2g carbohydrates, 24g fat, 1g fiber, 70mg cholesterol, 300mg sodium, 600mg potassium.*

Notes:
Salmon *is one of the best sources of omega-3 fatty acids, which have strong anti-inflammatory effects and support both heart and brain health. The addition of* **lemon** *not only adds a refreshing citrus flavor but also provides vitamin C, which boosts the immune system and enhances iron absorption.* **Thyme** *is known for its antioxidant properties, making this dish both delicious and beneficial for health.*

Tuna Tartare with Mango and Avocado
An exotic and nutritious dish, rich in antioxidants.

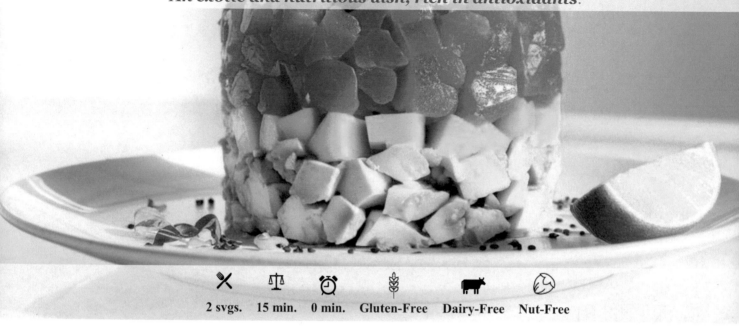

2 svgs.   **15 min.**   **0 min.**   **Gluten-Free**   **Dairy-Free**   **Nut-Free**

Ingredients:

- 6 oz fresh sushi-grade tuna, finely diced
- 1 small avocado, diced
- 1/2 cup fresh mango, diced
- 1 tbsp fresh lime juice
- 1 tsp sesame oil
- 1 tsp soy sauce (use gluten-free if needed)
- 1/2 tsp freshly grated ginger
- 1/2 tsp sea salt
- 1/4 tsp freshly ground black pepper
- 1 tbsp chopped fresh cilantro
- 1 tsp black sesame seeds (optional, for garnish)

Instructions:

1. In a medium bowl, combine the diced tuna, lime juice, sesame oil, soy sauce, grated ginger, sea salt, and black pepper. Mix gently until the tuna is well-coated with the marinade.
2. To assemble, place a layer of diced avocado at the bottom of a ring mold on a serving plate. Carefully add a layer of diced mango on top of the avocado.
3. Finally, add the marinated tuna mixture as the top layer. Carefully remove the ring mold to maintain the tartare's shape.
4. Garnish with chopped cilantro and black sesame seeds if desired. Serve immediately.

Nutrition Information: *280 calories, 20g protein, 12g carbohydrates, 18g fat, 5g fiber, 40mg cholesterol, 500mg sodium, 650mg potassium.*

Notes:

Tuna *is a rich source of omega-3 fatty acids, known for their powerful anti-inflammatory properties and for supporting both heart and brain health.* **Mango** *adds a sweet, tangy flavor along with a boost of vitamins A and C, both of which are important for immune function and skin health. Combined with the healthy fats from avocado, this tartare is not only delicious but also packed with nutrients that promote overall well-being.*

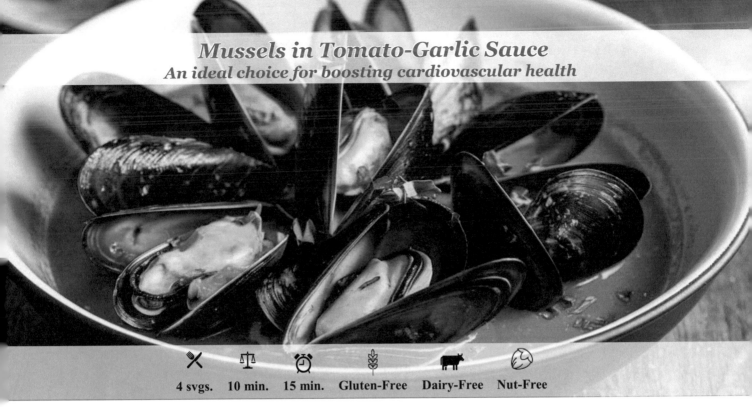

Mussels in Tomato-Garlic Sauce
An ideal choice for boosting cardiovascular health

4 svgs.   10 min.   15 min.   Gluten-Free   Dairy-Free   Nut-Free

Ingredients:

- 2 lbs fresh mussels, cleaned and debearded
- 1 tbsp olive oil
- 4 cloves garlic, minced
- 1 small onion, finely chopped
- 1 can (14.5 oz) diced tomatoes
- 1/4 cup dry white wine (optional)
- 1 tsp fresh thyme leaves (or 1/2 tsp dried thyme)
- 1/2 tsp sea salt
- 1/4 tsp freshly ground black pepper
- 1/4 tsp red pepper flakes (optional, for a spicy kick)
- Fresh parsley for garnish

Instructions:

1. Heat the olive oil in a large pot over medium heat. Add the chopped onion and garlic, and sauté until the onion is translucent and the garlic is fragrant, about 3-4 minutes.
2. Add the diced tomatoes, white wine (if using), thyme, sea salt, black pepper, and red pepper flakes. Bring the mixture to a simmer and cook for about 5 minutes, allowing the flavors to meld together.
3. Add the cleaned mussels to the pot, cover, and cook for 5-7 minutes, or until the mussels open up. Discard any mussels that do not open.
4. Serve the mussels hot, spooning the tomato-garlic sauce over them. Garnish with fresh parsley and serve with crusty bread or over pasta if desired.

Nutrition Information: *250 calories, 18g protein, 10g carbohydrates, 12g fat, 2g fiber, 50mg cholesterol, 600mg sodium, 800mg potassium.*

Notes:
__Mussels__ are an excellent source of high-quality protein and omega-3 fatty acids, which have anti-inflammatory properties and support heart health. __Tomatoes__ are rich in lycopene, a powerful antioxidant that helps reduce inflammation and supports skin health. This dish is not only delicious but also packed with nutrients that promote overall wellness.

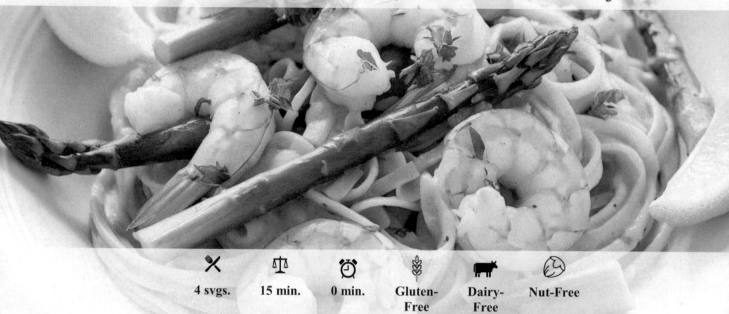

Shrimp and Asparagus Pasta in Light Lemon Sauce
Combines proteins and green vegetables for maximum health benefits.

✗	⚖	⏰	🌾	🐄	🌍
4 svgs.	15 min.	0 min.	Gluten-Free	Dairy-Free	Nut-Free

Ingredients:

- 8 oz gluten-free pasta (such as spaghetti or fettuccine)
- 1 lb large shrimp, peeled and deveined
- 1 bunch asparagus, trimmed and cut into 2-inch pieces
- 3 cloves garlic, minced
- 2 tbsp olive oil

- 1/4 cup fresh lemon juice
- Zest of 1 lemon
- 1/2 tsp sea salt
- 1/4 tsp freshly ground black pepper
- 1/4 cup fresh parsley, chopped
- Lemon wedges for serving (optional)

Instructions:

1. Cook the gluten-free pasta according to the package instructions until al dente. Drain and set aside.
2. While the pasta is cooking, heat 1 tablespoon of olive oil in a large skillet over medium heat. Add the asparagus and sauté for about 5 minutes, or until tender-crisp. Remove the asparagus from the skillet and set aside.
3. In the same skillet, add the remaining olive oil and minced garlic. Sauté for 1 minute until fragrant. Add the shrimp, sea salt, and black pepper, and cook until the shrimp are pink and opaque, about 3-4 minutes.
4. Add the cooked pasta, asparagus, lemon juice, and lemon zest to the skillet with the shrimp. Toss everything together until well combined and heated through.
5. Serve the pasta hot, garnished with chopped parsley and lemon wedges if desired.

Nutrition Information: 320 calories, 25g protein, 35g carbohydrates, 10g fat, 4g fiber, 150mg cholesterol, 450mg sodium, 500mg potassium

Notes:
Shrimp *are a great source of high-quality protein and omega-3 fatty acids, which help reduce inflammation and support heart health.* *Asparagus* *is rich in antioxidants, vitamins A, C, and E, and also has anti-inflammatory properties, making this dish both nutritious and delicious.*

Sea Bass Ceviche with Lime and Cilantro

A refreshing cold dish that helps maintain hydration and is packed with vitamins.

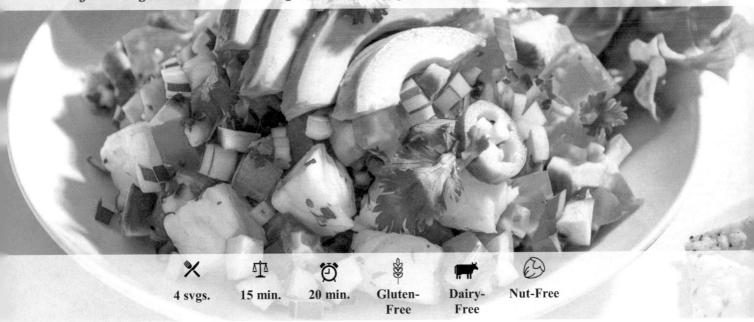

✕	⚖	⏰	🌾	🐄	🌐
4 svgs.	15 min.	20 min.	Gluten-Free	Dairy-Free	Nut-Free

Ingredients:

- 1 lb fresh sea bass fillet, diced into small cubes
- 1/2 cup fresh lime juice (about 4-5 limes)
- 1 small red onion, finely chopped
- 1 jalapeño pepper, seeded and finely chopped
- 1/2 cup fresh cilantro, chopped
- 1 small tomato, diced
- 1/4 cup cucumber, diced
- 1 avocado, diced
- 1 tsp sea salt
- 1/4 tsp freshly ground black pepper
- Tortilla chips or lettuce leaves for serving (optional)

Instructions:

1. In a medium glass or ceramic bowl, combine the diced sea bass and lime juice. Make sure the fish is fully submerged in the lime juice. Cover and refrigerate for 20 minutes, or until the fish turns opaque, indicating it is "cooked" by the acid in the lime juice.
2. Drain off most of the lime juice, leaving just a little to keep the fish moist. Add the chopped red onion, jalapeño, cilantro, tomato, cucumber, sea salt, and black pepper to the fish. Mix gently to combine.
3. Carefully fold in the diced avocado, trying not to mash it, and mix until everything is well combined.
4. Serve the ceviche immediately with tortilla chips or on lettuce leaves if desired.

Nutrition Information: 220 calories, 20g protein, 12g carbohydrates, 10g fat, 5g fiber, 50mg cholesterol, 400mg sodium, 600mg potassium

Notes:

Sea bass *is rich in lean protein and omega-3 fatty acids, which help reduce inflammation and support heart health?* **Lime** *juice is not only a key ingredient in ceviche but also a great source of vitamin C, which boosts the immune system and promotes healthy skin.* **Cilantro** *adds a burst of fresh flavor and contains antioxidants that further contribute to the anti-inflammatory benefits of this dish.*

Steamed Fish Fillet with Ginger and Green Onions

A light dish that preserves all the nutrients.

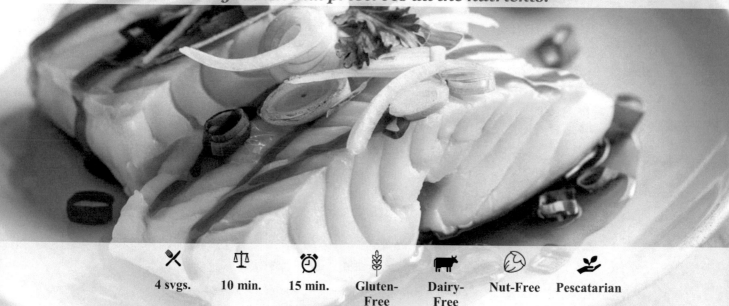

| 4 svgs. | 10 min. | 15 min. | Gluten-Free | Dairy-Free | Nut-Free | Pescatarian |

Ingredients:

- 4 fish fillets (such as cod, halibut, or sea bass), about 6 oz each
- 2 tbsp fresh ginger, julienned
- 4 green onions, cut into 2-inch pieces
- 2 tbsp soy sauce (use gluten-free if needed)
- 1 tbsp sesame oil
- 1 tbsp rice vinegar
- 1/4 tsp sea salt
- 1/4 tsp freshly ground black pepper
- 1 small bunch cilantro, chopped (optional, for garnish)
- Lemon or lime wedges for serving (optional)

Instructions:

1. Season the fish fillets with sea salt and black pepper on both sides. Set aside.
2. Prepare a steamer or place a steaming rack in a large pot filled with about 2 inches of water. Bring the water to a simmer.
3. Place the fish fillets on a heatproof plate that fits inside the steamer or pot. Sprinkle the julienned ginger and green onions evenly over the fish.
4. Steam the fish over simmering water for about 10-12 minutes, or until the fish is opaque and flakes easily with a fork.
5. While the fish is steaming, in a small bowl, mix together the soy sauce, sesame oil, and rice vinegar.
6. Once the fish is cooked, carefully remove it from the steamer and drizzle the soy sauce mixture over the fillets. Garnish with chopped cilantro and serve with lemon or lime wedges if desired.

Nutrition Information: 200 calories, 25g protein, 4g carbohydrates, 8g fat, 1g fiber, 55mg cholesterol, 500mg sodium, 400mg potassium

Notes:

Fish *like cod and halibut are rich in omega-3 fatty acids, which help reduce inflammation in the body. Ginger provides natural anti-inflammatory and antioxidant benefits, while green onions add vitamin C and antioxidants, supporting overall immune health. A light, nutritious dish that promotes well-being!*

Grilled Scallops with Blueberries and Mint

A unique flavor combination that promotes heart health.

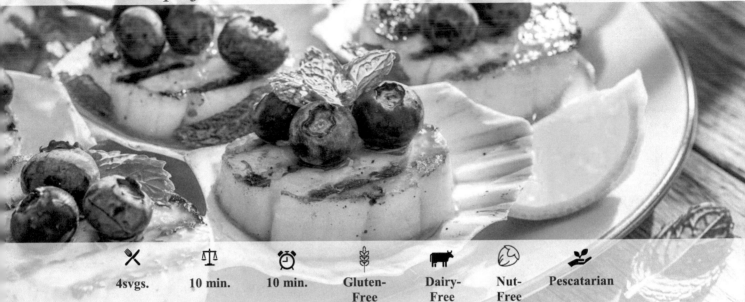

| 4svgs. | 10 min. | 10 min. | Gluten-Free | Dairy-Free | Nut-Free | Pescatarian |

Ingredients:

- 1 lb large sea scallops
- 2 tbsp olive oil
- 1 tbsp fresh lemon juice
- 1 tsp sea salt
- 1/4 tsp freshly ground black pepper
- 1 cup fresh blueberries
- 2 tbsp fresh mint leaves, chopped
- 1 tsp honey (optional)
- Lemon wedges for serving (optional)

Instructions:

1. Preheat your grill to medium-high heat. Pat the scallops dry with paper towels to remove any excess moisture.
2. In a small bowl, mix together the olive oil, lemon juice, sea salt, and black pepper. Brush the scallops with the mixture on both sides.
3. Grill the scallops for about 2-3 minutes per side, or until they are opaque and have nice grill marks. Be careful not to overcook them, as they can become tough.
4. While the scallops are grilling, prepare the blueberry-mint topping. In a small bowl, gently toss the fresh blueberries with chopped mint and honey if using.
5. Serve the grilled scallops hot, topped with the blueberry-mint mixture. Garnish with lemon wedges if desired.

Nutrition Information: 200 calories, 20g protein, 10g carbohydrates, 10g fat, 2g fiber, 40mg cholesterol, 500mg sodium, 300mg potassium

Notes:

Scallops are a great source of lean protein and omega-3 fatty acids, which help reduce inflammation and support heart health? **Blueberries** are packed with antioxidants, particularly anthocyanins, which have powerful anti-inflammatory effects. Combined with fresh mint, this dish offers a refreshing and nutritious balance that's perfect for a light, healthy meal.

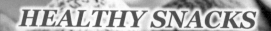

HEALTHY SNACKS

Nut and Date Energy Balls
A natural, portable energy boost that's easy to store and enjoy on the go.

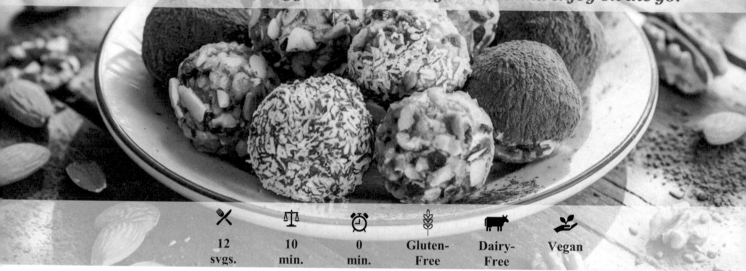

✕ 12 svgs.	⚖ 10 min.	⏰ 0 min.	🌾 Gluten-Free	🐄 Dairy-Free	🌱 Vegan

Ingredients:

- 1 cup Medjool dates, pitted
- 1/2 cup almonds (or sunflower seeds for nut-free option)
- 1/2 cup walnuts
- 1/4 cup shredded coconut (optional)
- 2 tbsp chia seeds
- 2 tbsp cocoa powder (optional, for a chocolate flavor)
- 1 tsp vanilla extract
- 1/4 tsp sea salt
- 1-2 tbsp water (if needed for consistency)

Instructions:

1. Prepare the Mixture: In a food processor, combine the pitted dates, almonds, walnuts, shredded coconut (if using), chia seeds, cocoa powder (if using), vanilla extract, and sea salt. Pulse until the mixture is finely ground and starts to stick together. Add water, if needed, one tablespoon at a time to achieve a sticky consistency.
2. Form the Balls: Scoop out a tablespoon-sized amount of the mixture and roll it between your hands to form a ball. Repeat with the remaining mixture.
3. Serve or Store: Serve the energy balls immediately or store them in an airtight container in the refrigerator for up to one week.

Nutrition Information: *120 calories, 3g protein, 12g carbohydrates, 7g fat, 3g fiber, 0mg cholesterol, 30mg sodium, 150mg potassium*

Notes:

Dates are naturally high in fiber and provide a quick source of energy, making them perfect for an on-the-go snack. **Nuts** like almonds and walnuts add healthy fats and protein, which help keep you satisfied and support brain health. These energy balls are a nutritious and delicious option to fuel your day.

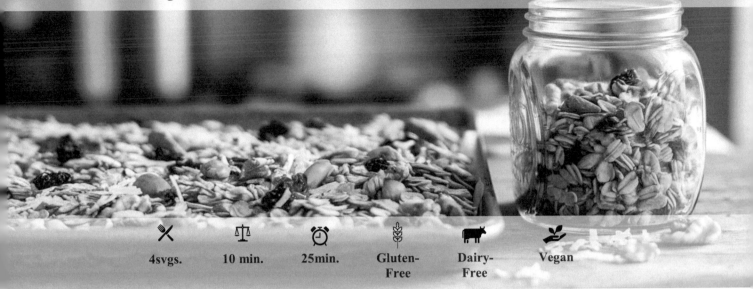

Homemade Granola
A healthy make-ahead option that adds variety to your breakfasts.

4svgs. | 10 min. | 25min. | Gluten-Free | Dairy-Free | Vegan

Ingredients:

- 3 cups old-fashioned rolled oats (gluten-free if needed)
- 1 cup chopped nuts (such as almonds, walnuts, or pecans)
- 1/2 cup unsweetened shredded coconut
- 1/4 cup chia seeds or flaxseeds (optional, for extra fiber)
- 1/2 cup dried fruit (such as cranberries, raisins, or chopped apricots)
- 1/3 cup coconut oil or olive oil, melted
- 1/3 cup maple syrup or honey
- 1 teaspoon vanilla extract
- 1/2 teaspoon ground cinnamon
- 1/4 teaspoon salt

Instructions:

1. Preheat Oven: Preheat your oven to 325°F (165°C). Line a large baking sheet with parchment paper.
2. Mix Dry Ingredients: In a large bowl, combine the oats, nuts, shredded coconut, chia seeds or flaxseeds (if using), cinnamon, and salt. Stir to combine.
3. Add Wet Ingredients: Pour the melted coconut oil, maple syrup or honey, and vanilla extract over the dry ingredients. Stir well until everything is evenly coated.
4. Bake the Granola: Spread the mixture evenly onto the prepared baking sheet. Bake for 20-25 minutes, stirring halfway through, until the granola is golden brown and fragrant. Keep an eye on it towards the end to avoid burning.
5. Cool and Add Dried Fruit: Remove the granola from the oven and let it cool completely on the baking sheet. Once cooled, stir in the dried fruit.
6. Serve Suggestions: Enjoy the granola on its own or serve it with yogurt, milk, or plant-based milk like almond or oat milk for a delicious and nutritious meal or snack.
7. Store: Transfer the granola to an airtight container and store it at room temperature for up to two weeks.

Nutritional Information (per 1/2 cup serving): *250 calories, 4g protein, 30g carbohydrates, 12g fats, 5g fiber, 0mg cholesterol, 75mg sodium, 150mg potassium.*

Notes: *Homemade granola allows you to control the ingredients, making it a healthier option compared to store-bought varieties. By using oats, nuts, and seeds, this granola is packed with fiber, healthy fats, and antioxidants, making it a perfect topping for smoothie bowls, yogurt parfaits, or just as a snack on its own.*

Apples with Almond Butter

A perfect blend of sweetness and protein, it's great for balancing blood sugar.

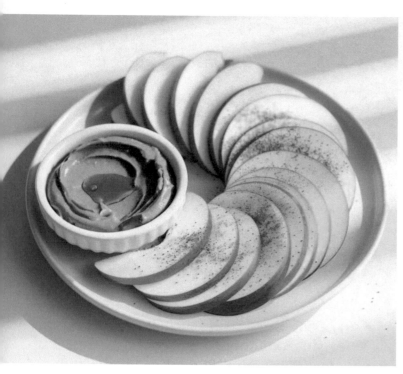

✕	⚖	⏰	🌾	🐄	🌱
2 svgs.	**5 min.**	**0 min.**	**Gluten-Free**	**Dairy-Free**	**Vegan**

Ingredients:

- 2 medium apples (such as Fuji, Gala, or Honeycrisp), cored and sliced
- 1/4 cup almond butter (or sunflower seed butter for a nut-free option)
- 1 tbsp honey or maple syrup (optional, for drizzling)
- 1 tbsp chia seeds (optional, for topping)
- 1/4 tsp ground cinnamon (optional, for dusting)

Instructions:

1. Prepare the Apples: Core and slice the apples into thin wedges. Arrange them on a serving plate.
2. Serve with Almond Butter: Serve the apple slices with almond butter on the side for dipping, or spread a little almond butter on each slice.
3. Add Optional Toppings: Drizzle with honey or maple syrup if desired. Sprinkle chia seeds and a dusting of ground cinnamon over the apple slices for added texture and flavor.
4. Serve: Enjoy immediately as a healthy snack or light dessert.

Nutrition Information: *180 calories, 3g protein, 24g carbohydrates, 10g fat, 4g fiber, 0mg cholesterol, 50mg sodium, 200mg potassium*

Notes:

Apples *are a great source of fiber, particularly pectin, which supports digestion and gut health, while their antioxidants help reduce inflammation.* *Almond butter* *provides healthy fats, protein, and vitamin E, an antioxidant that protects cells from damage.* *Chia seeds* *add omega-3 fatty acids, which are known for their anti-inflammatory benefits, and* *cinnamon* *helps regulate blood sugar and further boosts the dish's anti-inflammatory properties.*

This combination creates a balanced, nutrient-dense snack that's perfect for sustaining energy and supporting overall health.

Hummus with Carrot and Cucumber Sticks

An ideal source of protein and fiber, perfect for satisfying hunger.

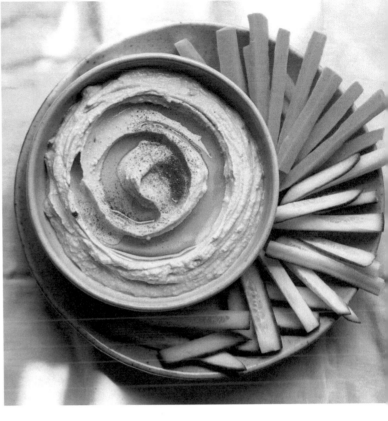

✕	⚖	⏰	🌾	🐄	🌍	🌱
4 svgs.	**15 min.**	**0 min.**	**Gluten-Free**	**Dairy-Free**	**Nut-Free**	**Vegan**

Ingredients:
For the Hummus:
- 1 can (15 oz) chickpeas, drained and rinsed
- 1/4 cup tahini
- 2 tbsp fresh lemon juice
- 2 cloves garlic, minced
- 2 tbsp olive oil
- 1/2 tsp sea salt
- 1/4 tsp ground cumin
- 1/4 cup cold water (or more for desired consistency)
- Paprika for garnish (optional)

For the Vegetable Sticks:
- 2 large carrots, peeled and cut into sticks
- 1 large cucumber, cut into sticks

Instructions:
1. Prepare the Hummus: In a food processor, combine the chickpeas, tahini, lemon juice, garlic, olive oil, sea salt, and cumin. Blend until smooth. Slowly add the cold water while blending until you reach your desired consistency. Adjust seasoning with more salt or lemon juice if needed.
2. Serve: Transfer the hummus to a serving bowl. Drizzle with a little olive oil and sprinkle with paprika if desired.
3. Prepare the Vegetable Sticks: Arrange the carrot and cucumber sticks around the hummus on a platter.
4. Serve: Serve immediately as a healthy snack or appetizer.

Nutrition Information: *180 calories, 6g protein, 15g carbohydrates, 10g fat, 5g fiber, 0mg cholesterol, 200mg sodium, 150mg potassium*

Notes:

Chickpeas, *the main ingredient in hummus, are rich in protein and fiber, which help promote digestive health and keep you feeling full longer.* **Tahini**, *made from sesame seeds, provides healthy fats and important minerals like calcium and magnesium. This combination makes hummus not only a delicious dip but also a nutritious snack that supports overall wellness.*

Vegetable Chips (Beet, Carrot, Zucchini)

A crispy and colorful snack that's both nutritious and delicious, perfect for satisfying your cravings without the guilt

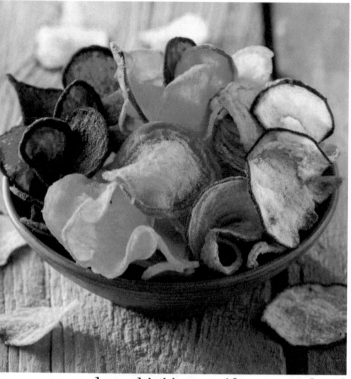

✖	⚖	⏰	🌾	🌍	🌱
4 svgs.	15 min.	25 min.	Gluten-Free	Nut-Free	Vegan

Ingredients:
- 1 large beet, peeled and thinly sliced
- 2 large carrots, peeled and thinly sliced
- 1 medium zucchini, thinly sliced
- 2 tbsp olive oil
- 1/2 tsp sea salt
- 1/4 tsp freshly ground black pepper
- 1/2 tsp smoked paprika (optional)

Instructions:
1. Preheat the Oven: Preheat your oven to 350°F (175°C). Line two baking sheets with parchment paper.
2. Prepare the Vegetables: Using a mandoline or a sharp knife, thinly slice the beet, carrots, and zucchini into uniform rounds. Place the sliced vegetables in a large bowl.
3. Season the Chips: Drizzle the olive oil over the sliced vegetables and toss to coat evenly. Sprinkle with sea salt, black pepper, and smoked paprika if using. Toss again to distribute the seasoning.
4. Bake the Chips: Arrange the vegetable slices in a single layer on the prepared baking sheets, making sure they do not overlap. Bake in the preheated oven for 20-25 minutes, flipping halfway through, until the chips are crispy and golden. Keep an eye on them to prevent burning, especially the thinner slices.
5. Cool and Serve: Remove the chips from the oven and let them cool completely on the baking sheets. They will continue to crisp up as they cool. Serve immediately or store in an airtight container for up to 3 days.

Nutrition Information: 100 calories, 2g protein, 12g carbohydrates, 5g fat, 3g fiber, 0mg cholesterol, 150mg sodium, 300mg potassium

Notes:
Beets are rich in antioxidants and nitrates, which help improve blood flow and lower blood pressure. *Carrots* provide beta-carotene, an antioxidant that supports vision and immune function. *Zucchini*, is a great source of vitamins C and B6, which support immune health and energy metabolism. These vegetable chips are a healthy alternative to traditional potato chips, offering both flavor and nutrition.

Greek Yogurt with Honey and Granola

Combines protein, probiotics, and carbohydrates for a balanced snack.

✗	⚖	⏰	🌾	🌍	🌿
2 svgs.	**5 min.**	**0 min.**	**Gluten -Free**	**Nut-Free**	**Vegeta rian**

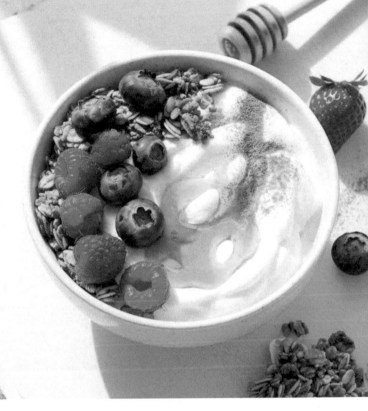

Ingredients:

- 1 cup Greek yogurt (plain or vanilla)
- 1/2 cup granola (use gluten-free or nut-free if needed)
- 2 tbsp honey
- 1/4 cup fresh berries (such as blueberries, strawberries, or raspberries)
- 1 tbsp chia seeds (optional, for topping)
- 1/2 tsp ground cinnamon (optional, for topping)

Instructions:

1. Prepare the Yogurt Base: Spoon the Greek yogurt into two serving bowls.
2. Add the Toppings: Drizzle 1 tablespoon of honey over each bowl of yogurt. Sprinkle 1/4 cup of granola over the top of each bowl.
3. Finish with Berries and Extras: Top with fresh berries and sprinkle with chia seeds and a dusting of ground cinnamon if desired.
4. Serve: Serve immediately as a nutritious breakfast or a healthy snack.

Nutrition Information: *200 calories, 10g protein, 30g carbohydrates, 6g fat, 4g fiber, 10mg cholesterol, 75mg sodium, 300mg potassium*

Notes:

Greek yogurt *is high in protein, which helps build and repair tissues and keeps you feeling full longer. It also contains probiotics, beneficial bacteria that support gut health.* **Honey** *provides natural sweetness and antioxidants, while granola adds a satisfying crunch and additional fiber. This combination makes for a delicious and balanced meal or snack that's both nutritious and satisfying.*

You can also experiment with seasonal fruits—try topping your yogurt with fresh berries in the summer, sliced apples or pears in the fall, or even pomegranate seeds in the winter. This dish is versatile and easily customizable, making it a perfect, balanced snack or breakfast option.

Oatmeal Bars with Blueberries and Nuts

A wholesome snack with a touch of crunch, packed with fiber, protein, and natural sweetness to keep you energized throughout the day.

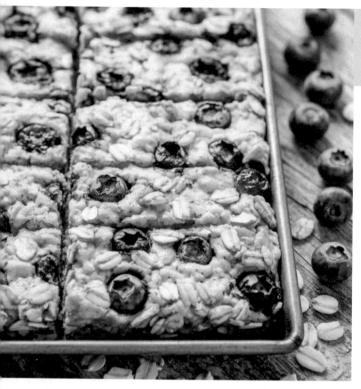

✗	⚖	⏰	🌾	🌱
8 svgs.	15 min.	25 min.	Gluten-Free	Vegetarian

Ingredients:

- 2 cups rolled oats (use gluten-free if needed)
- 1/2 cup almond flour (or sunflower seed flour for a nut-free option)
- 1/2 cup fresh or frozen blueberries
- 1/4 cup honey or maple syrup
- 1/4 cup coconut oil, melted
- 1/2 cup chopped nuts (such as almonds, walnuts, or pecans) or sunflower seeds
- 1/4 cup unsweetened applesauce
- 1 tsp vanilla extract
- 1/2 tsp ground cinnamon
- 1/4 tsp sea salt

Instructions:

1. Preheat the Oven: Preheat your oven to 350°F (175°C). Line an 8x8-inch baking pan with parchment paper, leaving some overhang for easy removal.
2. Prepare the Mixture: In a large bowl, combine the rolled oats, almond flour, chopped nuts or seeds, cinnamon, and sea salt. In a separate bowl, whisk together the melted coconut oil, honey or maple syrup, applesauce, and vanilla extract. Pour the wet ingredients into the dry ingredients and mix until well combined. Gently fold in the blueberries.
3. Form the Bars: Transfer the mixture to the prepared baking pan and press it down evenly with the back of a spoon or your hands to create a smooth, compact layer.
4. Bake: Bake in the preheated oven for 20-25 minutes, or until the edges are golden and the top is set. Remove from the oven and let cool completely in the pan on a wire rack.
5. Cut and Serve: Once cooled, lift the bars out of the pan using the parchment paper overhang and cut into 8 equal pieces. Serve immediately or store in an airtight container at room temperature for up to a week.

Nutrition Information: *200 calories, 4g protein, 24g carbohydrates, 10g fat, 3g fiber, 0mg cholesterol, 60mg sodium, 150mg potassium*

Notes:

Oats *are a great source of soluble fiber, particularly beta-glucan, which helps lower cholesterol levels and supports heart health.* **Blueberries** *are rich in antioxidants like vitamin C and anthocyanins, which have anti-inflammatory properties. These oatmeal bars provide a balanced mix of carbohydrates, healthy fats, and protein, making them a perfect on-the-go snack or a light breakfast option.*

Pumpkin Seed Crackers

Crunchy and savory, these crackers are packed with seeds and whole grains, providing a deliciously nutritious snack that's perfect on its own or paired with your favorite dips.

✕	⚖	⏰	🌾	🌍	🌱
8 svgs.	10 min.	25 min.	Gluten-Free	Nut-Free	Vegan

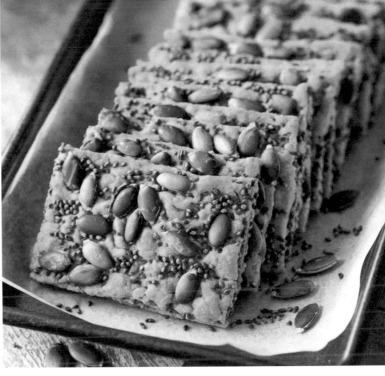

Ingredients:
- 1 cup pumpkin puree
- 1 cup rolled oats (use gluten-free if needed)
- 1/4 cup pumpkin seeds
- 1/4 cup sunflower seeds
- 2 tbsp flaxseed meal
- 1 tbsp chia seeds
- 1 tbsp olive oil
- 1/2 tsp sea salt
- 1/2 tsp ground cinnamon (optional)
- 1/4 tsp ground nutmeg (optional)

Instructions:
1. Preheat the Oven: Preheat your oven to 350°F (175°C). Line a baking sheet with parchment paper.
2. Prepare the Mixture: In a large bowl, combine the pumpkin puree, rolled oats, pumpkin seeds, sunflower seeds, flaxseed meal, chia seeds, olive oil, sea salt, ground cinnamon, and ground nutmeg (if using). Mix until all ingredients are well combined and form a thick dough.
3. Form the Crackers: Transfer the dough onto the prepared baking sheet. Use a spatula or your hands to spread the dough evenly into a thin layer, about 1/4 inch thick. To make it easier, you can place a piece of parchment paper on top of the dough and use a rolling pin to flatten it.
4. Score the Dough: Using a knife, score the dough into cracker-sized pieces to make it easier to break apart after baking.
5. Bake: Bake in the preheated oven for 20-25 minutes, or until the crackers are firm and the edges are lightly golden. Keep an eye on them to prevent burning.
6. Cool and Serve: Remove the baking sheet from the oven and let the crackers cool completely. Once cooled, break them into individual pieces along the scored lines. Serve immediately or store in an airtight container for up to one week.

Nutrition Information: *120 calories, 3g protein, 14g carbohydrates, 6g fat, 3g fiber, 0mg cholesterol, 90mg sodium, 200mg potassium*

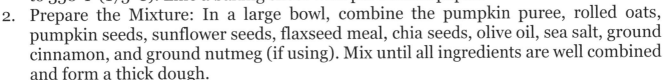

Notes:

Pumpkin is rich in vitamins A and C, both of which have antioxidant properties that help reduce inflammation. The addition of seeds like pumpkin, sunflower, and chia seeds adds healthy fats, protein, and fiber, making these crackers not only tasty but also a nutritious snack. Enjoy these crunchy, flavorful crackers on their own or with your favorite dip!

Crispy Chickpea Balls with Paprika

A crunchy, flavorful snack packed with protein and spices, perfect for a healthy bite any time of the day.

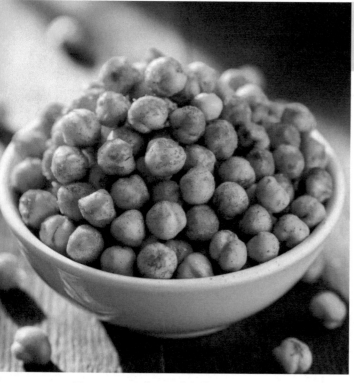

🍴	⚖️	⏰	🌾	🌍	🌱
4 svgs.	10 min.	25 min.	Gluten-Free	Nut-Free	Vegan

Ingredients:

- 1 can (15 oz) chickpeas, drained and rinsed
- 2 tbsp olive oil
- 1 tsp smoked paprika
- 1/2 tsp garlic powder
- 1/2 tsp onion powder
- 1/2 tsp sea salt
- 1/4 tsp freshly ground black pepper
- 1/4 tsp cayenne pepper (optional, for a spicy kick)

Instructions:

1. Preheat the Oven: Preheat your oven to 400°F (200°C). Line a baking sheet with parchment paper.
2. Prepare the Chickpeas: Pat the chickpeas dry with a clean kitchen towel or paper towel to remove excess moisture. This will help them get crispy in the oven.
3. Season the Chickpeas: In a large bowl, toss the chickpeas with olive oil, smoked paprika, garlic powder, onion powder, sea salt, black pepper, and cayenne pepper (if using). Make sure the chickpeas are evenly coated with the seasoning.
4. Bake the Chickpea Balls: Spread the seasoned chickpeas in a single layer on the prepared baking sheet. Bake in the preheated oven for 20-25 minutes, shaking the pan halfway through, until the chickpeas are golden and crispy.
5. Cool and Serve: Remove the chickpeas from the oven and let them cool slightly on the baking sheet. They will continue to crisp up as they cool. Serve warm or at room temperature as a crunchy snack.

Nutrition Information: *150 calories, 5g protein, 18g carbohydrates, 6g fat, 5g fiber, 0mg cholesterol, 300mg sodium, 200mg potassium*

Notes:

*Chickpeas are an excellent source of plant-based protein and fiber, which help maintain digestive health and keep you feeling full longer. The addition of smoked **paprika** provides a rich, smoky flavor, while **garlic and onion** powders add depth and complexity to the taste. These crispy chickpea balls are a perfect, healthy snack that's both delicious and satisfying.*

Avocado Toast on Whole Grain Bread

A rich source of healthy fats and fiber, perfect for a quick snack.

✗	⚖	⏰	🌑	🌱
2 svgs.	**10** min.	**0** min.	**Nut-Free**	**Vegan**

Ingredients:

- 2 slices whole grain bread (use gluten-free if needed)
- 1 large ripe avocado
- 1 tbsp fresh lemon juice
- 1/4 tsp sea salt
- 1/4 tsp freshly ground black pepper
- 1/4 tsp red pepper flakes (optional, for a bit of heat)
- 1/4 cup cherry tomatoes, halved
- 1 tbsp fresh cilantro or parsley, chopped
- 1 tbsp olive oil (optional, for drizzling)

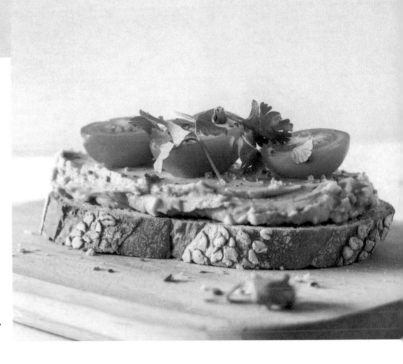

Instructions:

1. Prepare the Avocado Spread: Cut the avocado in half, remove the pit, and scoop the flesh into a bowl. Add the lemon juice, sea salt, and black pepper. Mash with a fork until smooth but still slightly chunky.
2. Assemble the Toast: Toast the whole grain bread slices to your desired level of crispiness. Spread the mashed avocado evenly over each slice of toast.
3. Add Toppings: Top the avocado spread with halved cherry tomatoes, a sprinkle of red pepper flakes (if using), and chopped fresh cilantro or parsley. Drizzle with olive oil for extra richness if desired.
4. Serve: Serve the avocado toast immediately, either on its own or with a side salad for a more substantial meal.

Nutrition Information: 250 calories, 5g protein, 22g carbohydrates, 16g fat, 7g fiber, 0mg cholesterol, 300mg sodium, 400mg potassium

Notes:

Avocados *are loaded with heart-healthy monounsaturated fats and fiber, which help keep you full and satisfied.* ***Whole grain bread*** *provides complex carbohydrates and additional fiber, contributing to better digestive health. This simple yet nutritious dish is perfect for a quick breakfast, lunch, or snack that's both delicious and good for you.*

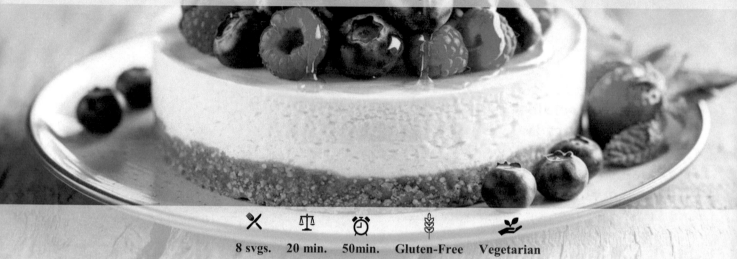

DIVINE DESSERTS

Almond Crust Cheesecake with Berries
A creamy, gluten-free dessert topped with fresh, antioxidant-rich berries.

8 svgs.   20 min.   50min.   Gluten-Free   Vegetarian

Ingredients:

For the Almond Crust:
- 1 1/2 cups almond flour
- 2 tbsp coconut sugar
- 1/4 cup melted coconut oil
- 1/2 tsp ground cinnamon (optional)
- 1/4 tsp sea salt

For the Cheesecake Filling:
- 16 oz (2 cups) cream cheese, softened
- 1/2 cup Greek yogurt
- 1/2 cup honey or maple syrup
- 2 large eggs
- 1 tsp vanilla extract
- 1 tbsp lemon juice

For the Berry Topping:
- 1 cup mixed fresh berries (such as strawberries, blueberries, raspberries)
- 1 tbsp honey or maple syrup (optional, for drizzling)
- Fresh mint leaves for garnish (optional)

Instructions:

1. Prepare the Almond Crust: Preheat your oven to 350°F (175°C). In a medium bowl, combine the almond flour, coconut sugar, melted coconut oil, ground cinnamon (if using), and sea salt. Mix until the ingredients are well combined and resemble a sandy texture. Press the mixture evenly into the bottom of a 9-inch springform pan to form the crust. Bake for 10 minutes, then set aside to cool.
2. Prepare the Cheesecake Filling: In a large bowl, beat the cream cheese until smooth and creamy. Add the Greek yogurt, honey or maple syrup, eggs, vanilla extract, and lemon juice. Beat until all ingredients are well combined and the mixture is smooth.
3. Bake the Cheesecake: Pour the cheesecake filling over the pre-baked almond crust, spreading it out evenly. Bake in the preheated oven for 40-45 minutes, or until the center is set but still slightly jiggly. Remove from the oven and let cool to room temperature, then refrigerate for at least 4 hours or overnight.
4. Add the Berry Topping: Before serving, top the chilled cheesecake with fresh mixed berries. Drizzle with honey or maple syrup if desired, and garnish with fresh mint leaves.
5. Serve: Slice and serve the cheesecake chilled. Store any leftovers in the refrigerator for up to 3 days.

Nutrition Information: *300 calories, 8g protein, 20g carbohydrates, 22g fat, 3g fiber, 80mg cholesterol, 200mg sodium, 150mg potassium*

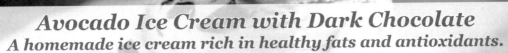

Avocado Ice Cream with Dark Chocolate
A homemade ice cream rich in healthy fats and antioxidants.

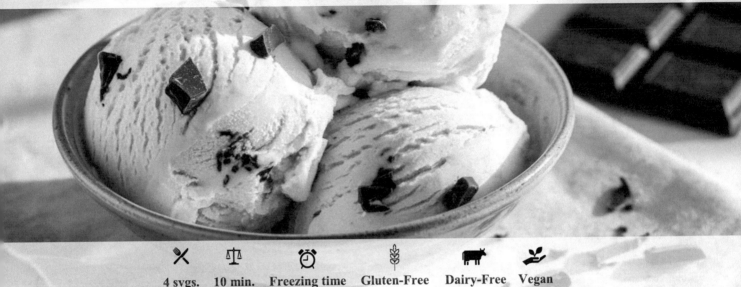

🍴	⚖️	⏰	🌾	🐄	🌱
4 svgs.	10 min.	Freezing time	Gluten-Free	Dairy-Free	Vegan

Ingredients:
- 2 ripe avocados, peeled and pitted
- 1/2 cup coconut milk (full-fat)
- 1/4 cup maple syrup or agave nectar
- 1 tbsp fresh lime juice
- 1 tsp vanilla extract
- 1/2 cup dark chocolate chips or chunks (dairy-free)

Instructions:
1. Blend the Base: In a blender or food processor, combine the avocados, coconut milk, maple syrup, lime juice, and vanilla extract. Blend until the mixture is smooth and creamy.
2. Add the Chocolate: Fold in the dark chocolate chips or chunks into the avocado mixture.
3. Freeze the Ice Cream: Transfer the mixture to a shallow, airtight container. Smooth the top with a spatula and cover with a lid or plastic wrap. Freeze for at least 4 hours or until firm.
4. Serve: Before serving, let the ice cream sit at room temperature for about 5-10 minutes to soften slightly. Scoop into bowls and enjoy!

Nutrition Information: *210 calories, 3g protein, 18g carbohydrates, 15g fat, 6g fiber, 0mg cholesterol, 20mg sodium, 400mg potassium*

Notes:
Avocados are rich in heart-healthy monounsaturated fats, which give the ice cream its smooth, velvety texture without the need for heavy cream. Pairing it with dark chocolate not only adds a deliciously rich flavor contrast, but also boosts the dessert's antioxidant content. Dark chocolate is known for its flavonoids, which help improve heart health and reduce inflammation. This unique combination makes avocado ice cream with dark chocolate a guilt-free indulgence that's both decadent and nutritious! For an extra twist, try sprinkling a pinch of sea salt or adding a few crushed pistachios for added crunch.

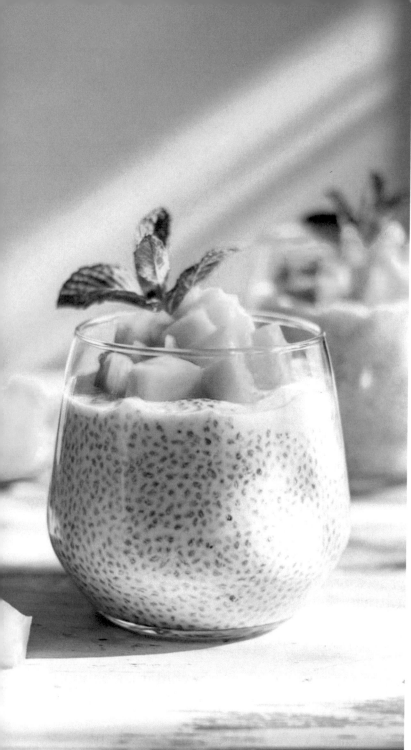

Coconut Pudding with Mango and Chia

A creamy, gluten-free dessert topped with fresh, antioxidant-rich berries.

✗	⚖	⏰	🌾	🌱
4svgs.	10 min.	Chilling time	Gluten -Free	Vegan

Ingredients:
- 1 can (14 oz) full-fat coconut milk
- 1/2 cup chia seeds
- 1/4 cup maple syrup or agave nectar
- 1 tsp vanilla extract
- 1 ripe mango, peeled and diced
- 1 tbsp fresh lime juice
- Fresh mint leaves for garnish (optional)

Instructions:
1. Prepare the Pudding Base: In a medium bowl, whisk together the coconut milk, chia seeds, maple syrup, and vanilla extract until well combined. Cover and refrigerate for at least 4 hours, or overnight, until the mixture thickens to a pudding-like consistency.
2. Prepare the Mango Topping: In a small bowl, toss the diced mango with fresh lime juice to enhance the flavor.
3. Assemble the Pudding: Spoon the thickened chia pudding into serving glasses or bowls. Top each serving with a generous amount of diced mango.
4. Garnish and Serve: Garnish with fresh mint leaves if desired. Serve chilled.

Nutrition Information: *250 calories, 4g protein, 28g carbohydrates, 15g fat, 8g fiber, 0mg cholesterol, 30mg sodium, 200mg potassium*

Notes:
Coconut pudding with mango and chia is not only a delicious tropical treat, but also a powerhouse of nutrients. **Coconut milk** provides healthy fats that help boost metabolism and keep you feeling satisfied. **Chia seeds** are rich in omega-3 fatty acids, fiber, and antioxidants, making them a perfect addition to this creamy dessert. **Mango** adds a burst of sweetness and vitamin C, supporting immune health and glowing skin. This pudding is not just a tasty indulgence, but also a nourishing option that's both refreshing and energizing. For extra flavor, try adding a squeeze of lime juice or a sprinkle of toasted coconut on top!

Pumpkin Mousse with Coconut Cream

A seasonal dessert with low sugar content, rich in vitamins A and C.

 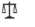

| 4svgs | 15 min. | Chilling time. | Gluten-Free | Nut-Free | Vegan |

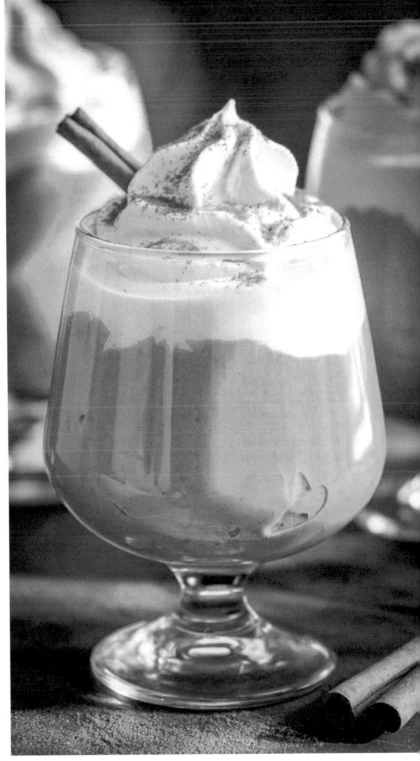

Ingredients:

For the Pumpkin Mousse:

- 1 cup pumpkin puree
- 1/2 cup coconut milk (full-fat)
- 1/4 cup maple syrup or agave nectar
- 1 tsp vanilla extract
- 1/2 tsp ground cinnamon
- 1/4 tsp ground nutmeg
- 1/8 tsp ground ginger
- 1/8 tsp ground cloves (optional)

For the Coconut Cream:

- 1 can (14 oz) coconut cream, chilled overnight
- 2 tbsp powdered sugar or maple syrup
- 1/2 tsp vanilla extract

Instructions:

1. Prepare the Pumpkin Mousse: In a large mixing bowl, combine the pumpkin puree, coconut milk, maple syrup, vanilla extract, ground cinnamon, nutmeg, ginger, and cloves (if using). Whisk until the mixture is smooth and well combined. Refrigerate for at least 1 hour to let the flavors meld and the mousse thickens slightly.
2. Prepare the Coconut Cream: Open the chilled can of coconut cream and scoop out the thick, solid cream into a mixing bowl (leave any liquid behind). Add the powdered sugar or maple syrup and vanilla extract. Use an electric mixer to whip the coconut cream until it becomes light and fluffy, about 2-3 minutes.
3. Assemble the Mousse: Spoon the pumpkin mousse into serving glasses or bowls. Top each serving with a generous dollop of whipped coconut cream.
4. Serve: Garnish with a sprinkle of ground cinnamon or a cinnamon stick for an extra touch. Serve chilled and enjoy!

Nutrition Information: *200 calories, 2g protein, 18g carbohydrates, 14g fat, 3g fiber, 0mg cholesterol, 10mg sodium, 150mg potassium*

Carob Brownies with Nuts
A great alternative to traditional chocolate brownies.

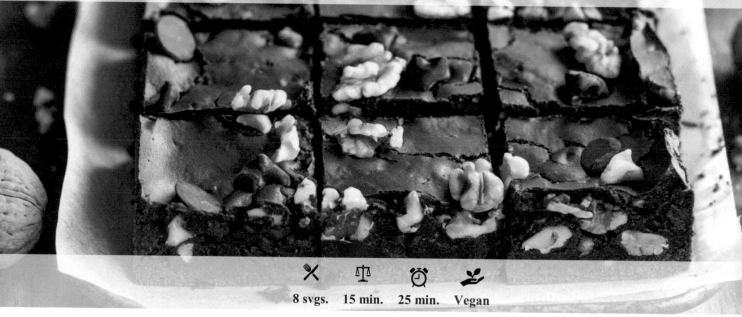

8 svgs.   15 min.   25 min.   Vegan

Ingredients:

- 1/2 cup carob powder
- 1 cup gluten-free flour blend (or regular flour)
- 1/2 cup coconut sugar
- 1/2 cup coconut oil, melted
- 1/4 cup almond milk (or any plant-based milk)

- 1 tsp vanilla extract
- 1/2 tsp baking powder
- 1/4 tsp sea salt
- 1/2 cup chopped walnuts (or sunflower seeds for nut-free option)
- 1/4 cup dairy-free chocolate chips (optional)

Instructions:

1. Preheat the Oven: Preheat your oven to 350°F (175°C). Line an 8x8-inch baking pan with parchment paper, leaving some overhang for easy removal.
2. Prepare the Brownie Batter: In a large bowl, whisk together the carob powder, gluten-free flour, coconut sugar, baking powder, and sea salt. In a separate bowl, mix the melted coconut oil, almond milk, and vanilla extract. Pour the wet ingredients into the dry ingredients and stir until just combined. Fold in the chopped walnuts and dairy-free chocolate chips (if using).
3. Bake the Brownies: Pour the batter into the prepared baking pan, spreading it out evenly. Bake in the preheated oven for 20-25 minutes, or until a toothpick inserted into the center comes out clean or with a few moist crumbs.
4. Cool and Serve: Allow the brownies to cool completely in the pan on a wire rack. Once cooled, lift the brownies out of the pan using the parchment paper overhang and cut into 8 equal pieces. Serve immediately or store in an airtight container at room temperature for up to 3 days.

Nutrition Information: *210 calories, 4g protein, 24g carbohydrates, 12g fat, 3g fiber, 0mg cholesterol, 80mg sodium, 150mg potassium*

Notes:
Carob is a natural, caffeine-free alternative to cocoa powder and is rich in fiber and antioxidants, which help reduce inflammation and support heart health. Adding nuts like walnuts provides healthy fats and additional protein, making these brownies not only delicious but also nutritious.

Almond Truffles with Dark Chocolate
Indulgent bite-sized treats featuring a rich dark chocolate coating and a creamy almond center.

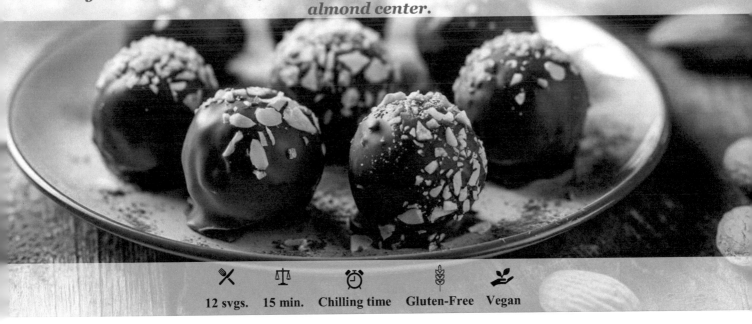

12 svgs.   **15 min.**   **Chilling time**   **Gluten-Free**   **Vegan**

Ingredients:
- 1 cup almond flour
- 1/4 cup cocoa powder (unsweetened)
- 1/4 cup maple syrup or agave nectar
- 1/4 cup almond butter (or any nut butter of choice)
- 1 tsp vanilla extract
- 1/4 tsp sea salt
- 1/2 cup dark chocolate chips (dairy-free)
- 1 tbsp coconut oil
- 1/4 cup crushed almonds (for rolling, optional)

Instructions:
1. Prepare the Truffle Base: In a medium bowl, combine the almond flour, cocoa powder, maple syrup, almond butter, vanilla extract, and sea salt. Mix until all ingredients are well combined and form a thick, dough-like consistency.
2. Form the Truffles: Using a tablespoon, scoop out portions of the mixture and roll them into small balls with your hands. Set the balls on a parchment-lined tray or plate.
3. Melt the Chocolate: In a microwave-safe bowl, combine the dark chocolate chips and coconut oil. Microwave in 20-second intervals, stirring between each, until the chocolate is fully melted and smooth.
4. Coat the Truffles: Dip each truffle ball into the melted chocolate, using a fork to roll it around until fully coated. Allow any excess chocolate to drip off before placing the truffle back on the parchment paper. Optionally, roll the coated truffles in crushed almonds for added texture.
5. Chill and Serve: Place the truffles in the refrigerator for about 20-30 minutes, or until the chocolate coating is set. Serve chilled or at room temperature.

Nutrition Information: *120 calories, 3g protein, 10g carbohydrates, 8g fat, 2g fiber, 0mg cholesterol, 30mg sodium, 80mg potassium*

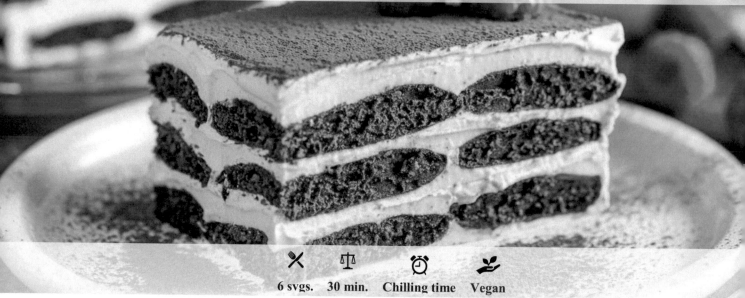

Vegan Tiramisu with Cashew Cream
A rich, dairy-free dessert that will satisfy any coffee dessert lover.

6 svgs.   30 min.   Chilling time   Vegan

Ingredients:

For the Cashew Cream:
- 1 cup raw cashews, soaked for at least 4 hours or overnight
- 1/2 cup coconut cream
- 1/4 cup maple syrup
- 2 tbsp lemon juice
- 1 tsp vanilla extract

For the Coffee Soak:
- 1 cup strong brewed coffee, cooled
- 2 tbsp coffee liqueur (optional)

- 1 tbsp maple syrup

For the Assembly:
- 12-15 gluten-free vegan ladyfingers or sponge cake slices
- 2 tbsp cocoa powder (for dusting)
- Fresh raspberries or strawberries for garnish (optional)
- Fresh mint leaves for garnish (optional)

Instructions:

1. Prepare the Cashew Cream: Drain and rinse the soaked cashews. In a high-speed blender, combine the cashews, coconut cream, maple syrup, lemon juice, and vanilla extract. Blend until smooth and creamy, scraping down the sides as needed. Set aside.
2. Prepare the Coffee Soak: In a shallow dish, mix the brewed coffee, coffee liqueur (if using), and maple syrup. Stir to combine.
3. Assemble the Tiramisu: Dip each ladyfinger or sponge cake slice briefly into the coffee soak, making sure both sides are moistened but not soggy. Arrange a layer of soaked ladyfingers at the bottom of a 9x9-inch dish or individual serving glasses. Spread half of the cashew cream evenly over the soaked ladyfingers.
4. Repeat Layers: Repeat the process with another layer of soaked ladyfingers and the remaining cashew cream. Smooth the top layer with a spatula.
5. Chill and Serve: Cover and refrigerate for at least 4 hours or overnight to let the flavors meld and the dessert to set. Before serving, dust the top with cocoa powder and garnish with fresh raspberries or strawberries and mint leaves if desired.

Nutrition Information: 320 calories, 6g protein, 30g carbohydrates, 20g fat, 4g fiber, 0mg cholesterol, 15mg sodium, 200mg potassium

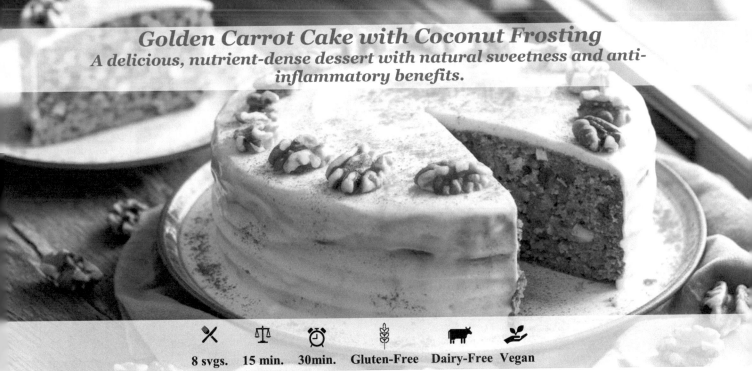

Golden Carrot Cake with Coconut Frosting

A delicious, nutrient-dense dessert with natural sweetness and anti-inflammatory benefits.

🍴 8 svgs.　⚖️ 15 min.　⏰ 30min.　🌾 Gluten-Free　🐄 Dairy-Free　🌱 Vegan

Ingredients:

For the Cake:

- 2 cups grated carrots
- 1 1/2 cups almond flour
- 1/2 cup oat flour (gluten-free if needed)
- 1/4 cup coconut sugar or maple syrup
- 1/4 cup coconut oil, melted
- 1/4 cup unsweetened applesauce
- 2 tsp ground cinnamon
- 1 tsp ground ginger
- 1/4 tsp ground turmeric (optional, for extra anti-inflammatory boost)
- 1 tsp baking soda
- 1/4 tsp sea salt
- 1 tsp vanilla extract
- 1/4 cup chopped walnuts or pecans (optional)

For the Frosting:

- 1 cup coconut yogurt or cashew cream
- 2 tbsp maple syrup or honey
- 1 tsp vanilla extract
- 1/2 tsp ground cinnamon

Instructions:

1. Preheat the Oven: Preheat your oven to 350°F (175°C) and line an 8-inch cake pan with parchment paper or lightly grease it with coconut oil.
2. Mix the Dry Ingredients: In a large bowl, whisk together almond flour, oat flour, coconut sugar, cinnamon, ginger, turmeric (if using), baking soda, and sea salt.
3. Mix the Wet Ingredients: In a separate bowl, combine melted coconut oil, applesauce, vanilla extract, and grated carrots.
4. Combine and Add Nuts: Slowly add the wet ingredients to the dry ingredients and stir until well combined. Fold in the chopped walnuts or pecans if desired.
5. Bake the Cake: Pour the batter into the prepared cake pan and smooth the top. Bake for 25-30 minutes, or until a toothpick inserted into the center comes out clean. Let the cake cool completely before frosting.
6. Prepare the Frosting: In a small bowl, whisk together coconut yogurt (or cashew cream), maple syrup, vanilla extract, and cinnamon until smooth.
7. Frost and Serve: Once the cake has cooled, spread the frosting evenly on top. Slice and serve!

Nutrition Information: *200 calories, 5g protein, 18g carbohydrates, 14g fat, 4g fiber, 0mg cholesterol, 70mg sodium, 300mg potassium*

30-Day Meal Plan

Day	Breakfast	Lunch	Dinner	Snack
Day 1	Veggie-Stuffed Omelet	Sweet Potato Soup with Ginger and Coconut Milk	Spinach and Feta Stuffed Turkey Brea and Kale and Pomegranate Salad with Tahini Dressing	Nut and Date Energy Balls
Day 2	Broccoli and Bell Pepper Frittata	Rosemary and Lemon Baked Chicken Breast and Burrata, Basil, and Tomato Salad	Niçoise Salad with Tuna and Egg	Homemade Granola with coconut milk
Day 3	Acai Smoothie Bowl	Chicken Vegetable Soup with Thyme	Grilled Salmon with Lemon-Thyme Marinade and Greek Salad with Olives and Feta	Apples with Almond Butter
Day 4	Green Smoothie with Spinach, Avocado, and Kiwi	Turkish Meatballs with Cilantro and Mint and Artichoke, Pepper, and Arugula Salad	Quinoa Salad with Avocado and Cherry Tomatoes	Hummus with Carrot and Cucumber Sticks
Day 5	Berry Chia Oatmeal with Old-Fashioned Oats	Creamy Broccoli Soup with Almond Milk	Turkey with Cranberry Sauce and Quinoa	Vegetable Chips (Beet, Carrot, Zucchini)
Day 6	Buckwheat Pancakes with Apple Sauce	Duck with Orange Sauce and Thyme and Kale and Pomegranate Salad with Tahini Dressing	Chicken Caesar Salad with Homemade Croutons	Greek Yogurt with Honey and Granola
Day 7	Avocado and Salmon Toast	Tomato Soup with Basil and Garlic and Chicken Marsala with Mushrooms	Avocado and Salmon Salad	Oatmeal Bars with Blueberries and Nuts
Day 8	Berry and Nut Yogurt Parfait with Honey	Honey Mustard Chicken Wings and Greek Salad with Olives and Feta	Shrimp and Asparagus Pasta in Light Lemon Sauce	Pumpkin Seed Crackers
Day 9	Quinoa Porridge with Almond Milk and Cinnamon	Lentil Soup with Turmeric and Spinach	Sea Bass Ceviche with Lime and Cilantro	Crispy Chickpea Balls with Paprika
Day 10	Chia Pudding with Mango and Coconut	Asian-Style Chicken with Ginger and Soy Sauce and Sweet Potato, Cilantro, and Black Bean Salad	Grilled Scallops with Blueberries and Mint and Artichoke, Pepper, and Arugula Salad	Avocado Toast on Whole Grain Bread
Day 11	Veggie-Stuffed Omelet	Seafood Broth with Fennel and Celery	Spinach and Feta Stuffed Turkey Breast served with a side of seasonal vegetable slices.	Coconut Pudding with Mango and Chia

Day 12	Broccoli and Bell Pepper Frittata	Chicken Marsala with Mushrooms served with a garnish of your choice	Steamed Fish Fillet with Ginger and Green Onions and Kale and Pomegranate Salad with Tahini Dressing	Carob Brownies with Nuts
Day 13	Acai Smoothie Bowl	Miso Soup with Tofu and Seaweed and Tuna Tartare with Mango and Avocado	Honey Mustard Chicken Wings and Beet Salad with Goat Cheese and Pecans	Almond Truffles with Dark Chocolate
Day 14	Green Smoothie with Spinach, Avocado, and Kiwi	Grilled Salmon with Lemon-Thyme Marinade and Greek Salad with Olives and Feta	Chicken Caesar Salad with Homemade Croutons	Pumpkin Mousse with Coconut Cream
Day 15	Berry Chia Oatmeal with Old-Fashioned Oats	Mushroom, Thyme, and Garlic Soup	Asian-Style Chicken with Ginger and Soy Sauce and Sweet Potato, Cilantro, and Black Bean Salad	Nut and Date Energy Balls
Day 16	Buckwheat Pancakes with Apple Sauce	Sweet Potato Soup with Ginger and Coconut Milk	Spinach and Feta Stuffed Turkey Brea and Kale and Pomegranate Salad with Tahini Dressing	Homemade Granola with coconut milk
Day 17	Avocado and Salmon Toast	Rosemary and Lemon Baked Chicken Breast and Artichoke, Pepper, and Arugula Salad	Niçoise Salad with Tuna and Egg	Apples with Almond Butter
Day 18	Berry and Nut Yogurt Parfait with Honey	Chicken Vegetable Soup with Thyme	Grilled Salmon with Lemon-Thyme Marinade and Greek Salad with Olives and Feta	Hummus with Carrot and Cucumber Sticks
Day 19	Quinoa Porridge with Almond Milk and Cinnamon	Turkish Meatballs with Cilantro and Mint and Burrata, Basil, and Tomato Salad	Quinoa Salad with Avocado and Cherry Tomatoes	Vegetable Chips (Beet, Carrot, Zucchini)
Day 20	Chia Pudding with Mango and Coconut	Creamy Broccoli Soup with Almond Milk	Turkey with Cranberry Sauce and Quinoa	Greek Yogurt with Honey and Granola
Day 21	Veggie-Stuffed Omelet	Duck with Orange Sauce and Thyme and Greek Salad with Olives and Feta	Chicken Caesar Salad with Homemade Croutons	Oatmeal Bars with Blueberries and Nuts
Day 22	Broccoli and Bell Pepper Frittata	Tomato Soup with Basil and Garlic and Chicken Marsala with Mushrooms	Avocado and Salmon Salad	Pumpkin Seed Crackers
Day 23	Acai Smoothie Bowl	Honey Mustard Chicken Wings and Kale and Pomegranate Salad with Tahini Dressing	Shrimp and Asparagus Pasta in Light Lemon Sauce	Crispy Chickpea Balls with Paprika
Day 24	Green Smoothie with Spinach, Avocado, and Kiwi	Lentil Soup with Turmeric and Spinach	Turkey with Cranberry Sauce and Quinoa	Avocado Toast on Whole Grain Bread

Day 25	Berry Chia Oatmeal with Old-Fashioned Oats	Asian-Style Chicken with Ginger and Soy Sauce and Greek Salad with Olives and Feta	Grilled Scallops with Blueberries and Mint and Artichoke, Pepper, and Arugula Salad	Coconut Pudding with Mango and Chia
Day 26	Buckwheat Pancakes with Apple Sauce	Seafood Broth with Fennel and Celery	Spinach and Feta Stuffed Turkey Breast served with a side of seasonal vegetable slices.	Carob Brownies with Nuts
Day 27	Avocado and Salmon Toast	Chicken Marsala with Mushrooms served with a garnish of your choice	Steamed Fish Fillet with Ginger and Green Onions and Kale and Pomegranate Salad with Tahini Dressing	Almond Truffles with Dark Chocolate
Day 28	Berry and Nut Yogurt Parfait with Honey	Miso Soup with Tofu and Seaweed and Tuna Tartare with Mango and Avocado	Honey Mustard Chicken Wings and Beet Salad with Goat Cheese and Pecans	Pumpkin Mousse with Coconut Cream
Day 29	Quinoa Porridge with Almond Milk and Cinnamon	Grilled Salmon with Lemon-Thyme Marinade and Sweet Potato, Cilantro, and Black Bean Salad	Chicken Caesar Salad with Homemade Croutons	Green Smoothie with Spinach, Avocado, and Kiwi
Day 30	Chia Pudding with Mango and Coconut	Mushroom, Thyme, and Garlic Soup	Asian-Style Chicken with Ginger and Soy Sauce and Greek Salad with Olives and Feta	Homemade Granola with Almond milk

Friendly reminder: While we've included the nutritional values for the dishes in our book, please note these are estimates. For precise nutritional information, calculate based on the specific brands and quantities of ingredients you use.

Happy cooking!

Made in the USA
Columbia, SC
23 December 2024

50588338R00048